CHINESE
HERBAL MEDICINE

THE KEY TO HEALTH
AND WELL-BEING

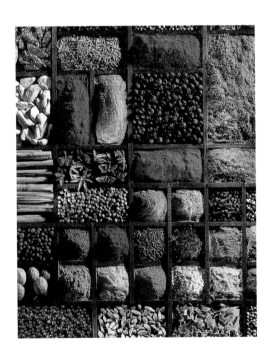

Important

This book has been researched in accordance with the most recent information.
Nevertheless, all information is supplied without liability.
The publisher can except no responsibility for potential detriment and injury,
which result from following the practical advice in this book.
The pieces of advise contained in this book do not replace the examination and care given by a doctor.
Before carrying out a treatment on yourself, you should consult a doctor,
especially if you suffer from a health complaint, take regular medication or are pregnant.

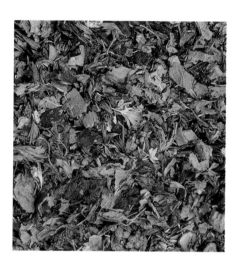

List of picture sources:

Bavaria, Dusseldorf: 1, 4, 5, 8, 12, 13, 14, 19, 21, 22, 23, 24, 25 bottom, 26, 27 bottom left,
31, 35, 36, 37, 42, 46, 50 top, 60, 61
Fotodienst Fehn, Lage: 39, 41 43, 47, 48, 53 top
MEV, Augsburg: 2, 10, 11 right, 15, 16, 17, 20, 27 top left, 27 top right, 32 bottom, 34, 38, 44, 54, 55,
miniatures 4, 10-28, 34-38, 62-64
PhotoPress, Stockdorf/Munich: 11 left, 25 top, 27 bottom right, 28, 33
Foto Reinhard, Heiligkreuzsteinach: 6, 40, 45, 50 bottom, 51, 53 bottom, 57 bottom, 58, 59, 62
VEMAG, Cologne: 29, 30, 32 top, 49, 52, 56, 57 top, miniatures 5-9, 29-33, 39-61

Chinese Herbal Medicine

© Neuer Pawlak Verlag
Part of the VEMAG Verlags- und Medien Aktiengesellschaft, Cologne
Author: Georgia Schwarz
Cover: Jump, Hamburg
Produced by: Neuer Pawlak Verlag, Cologne
All rights reserved

ISBN 3-86146-029-7

CONTENTS

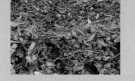

FOREWORD

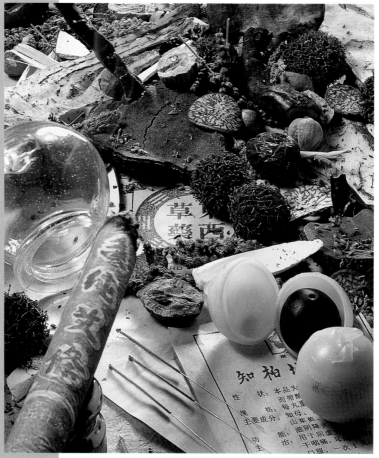

Thousands of years ago in ancient China, it was considered a human right to protect your body through conscious healthy living. Ancient Chinese healing experts recognised early on that a healthy mind is a prerequisite for a healthy body, since both are inseparable.

This knowledge is no longer present in today's high-tech world. Complicated treatments, which are often biased and accompanied by numerous side effects, are the results of over-specialised western medicine.

Chinese herbal medicine, which is seen as an integral medicine, presents itself as a useful supplement to the western view of medicine, because the whole body is taken into consideration for diagnosis and treatment.

This book is here to help you use the knowledge of this alternative medicine for your own health.

After an introduction into the basics and the way of thinking in Chinese medicine, you will receive simple recommendations for a healthy way of living and a balanced diet, which touch on knowledge acquired centuries ago. A detailed herbal study in the second part of this book shows that at least one Chinese herb grows for nearly every illness. Naturally, we have only considered such herbs and remedies that are available in our western society here in this book.

At the end of this book, you will find useful addresses of chemists and companies, who can help you to obtain literature or rare Chinese herbs, if you wish to find out more about this fascinating alternative medicine.

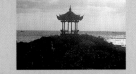

THE HISTORY OF TRADITIONAL CHINESE MEDICINE

Protecting your body through a healthy way of living is one of the fundamental teachings of Chinese medicine, also recognised 2000 years ago by Confucius. "You should not do anything that could harm your body, not even to your skin or hair, because you inherit them from your father and mother". This is one of his basic rules.

The first famous doctor of the Chinese classical antiquity was Bianque, who lived about 500 AD. He was allegedly the founder of acupuncture and pulse diagnoses. Besides this he is also the inventor of different diagnosis methods, for example "listening to breathing", the examination of the facial colour and the questioning of patients, which corresponds to today's examinations. Supposedly he could bring people who were taken for dead, back to life. This should not be taken literally.

The lessons of various ancient Chinese philosophers filtered into traditional Chinese medicine. Depending upon the evaluation, interpretation or translation of these lessons, over the years various schools of Chinese medicine were developed and with this the medicine became unclear. That is why in the second half of the 7th century, Liu Yuansu cut back the collected works of over 16 000 remedies to around 300.

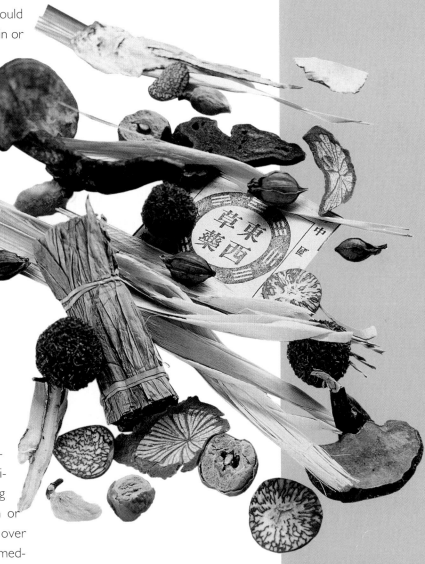

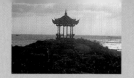

TRADITIONAL CHINESE MEDICINE

Besides this, he classified the various types of illnesses, into six different categories, they differentiate on the basis of the five elements – water, fire, wood, metal and earth. Through these measures the traditional Chinese medicine was made considerably simpler.

The classic work of Chinese pharmaceutical is "Bencao gangmu", ("The Register of Medical Matter") by Li Shizhen. He lived from 1518 to 1593. The study embraces three categories herbs, animals and minerals, and is divided into 16 chapters with 62 subchapters. In this book you will find more than 1,000 illustrations and over 10,000 remedies. It has been completely revised three times and translated into many languages. It is still published to this day.

Over the last thousands of years many treatments have developed in traditional Chinese medicine that can be used on their own or in combination with others. Belonging to these, are for instance, acupressure, acupuncture, acupunct-massage, diet council, harmony study and the decorating art of Feng Shui, herbal medicine, qi gong (meditation) and tai chi (movement and breathing therapy).

For years the traditional Chinese medicine has been categorised as superstitious, even the simple full body diagnosis and the acupuncture technique were misunderstood and misjudged, because they could not withstand the standards of the western world. They did not correspond with our medical demands of objectivity and examination. Yet since then, European and also British doctors have, after the initial scepticism, confirmed the effect of traditional Chinese treatments. In China, traditional Chinese medicine is used mainly for simple complaints, functional disturbances and for chronic illnesses.

The illustration shows a memorial for the Chinese pharmacist Li Shizhen.

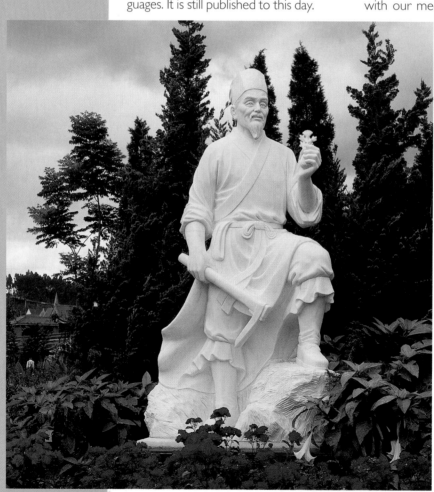

THE PRINCIPLE OF YIN AND YANG

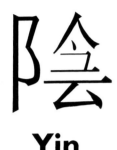

Yin

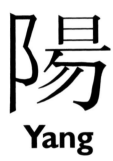

Yang

and the never-ending process of natural change.

It is interesting here to examine the Chinese character for Yin and Yang.

The oldest fundamental idea of Chinese philosophy, which also shows itself in all departments of science and therefore also in medicine, is the concept of two opposite poles: Yin and Yang. Symbolically Yin and Yang are depicted as two embracing fish, which together create a whole. Yin and Yang originate out of a whole or out of nothing. From them all things in the universe are created.

With both these fundamental concepts Chinese philosophy explains relationships of every being to each other – whether living or inanimate – but also to the universe

The Manifestations of Yin and Yang

Yin is dark	Yang is light
Yin is green, blue, black, brown	Yang is red, orange, yellow
Yin is still	Yang is moving
Yin is contracting	Yang is expansive
Yin is angular	Yang is round but not circular
Yin is narrow	Yang is wide
Yin is slow	Yang is fast
Yin is passive	Yang is active
Yin is earth	Yang is sky
Yin is water	Yang is mountains
Yin is moon	Yang is sun
Yin is rain	Yang is sunshine
Yin is odd numbers	Yang is even numbers
Yin is winter	Yang is summer
Yin is coolness	Yang is warmth
Yin is tiger	Yang is dragon
Yin is below	Yang is above
Yin is deep	Yang is high
Yin is downwards	Yang is upwards
Yin is soft	Yang is hard
Yin is cold	Yang is hot
Yin is woman	Yang is man
Yin is ground	Yang is peak
Yin is sour	Yang is sweet
Yin is sad	Yang is angry
Yin is shadow	Yang is light
Yin is night	Yang is day

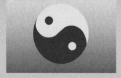

The following body parts are divided into Yin and Yang categories:

Yin	Yang
Stomache	Back
Legs	Arms
Blood	Energy (Qi)

They consist of various signs. The character for Yin consists of the signs for a hill, a cloud and many people who gather in a group under one roof. Yin has characteristics such as cold, peace, receptiveness, passiveness, darkness, reduction, the inner being as well as the direction below and downwards.

The character for Yang consists of the signs for a hill, the sun over the horizon as well as light beams, and for moving energy. Consequently Yang has characteristics such as heat, movement, activity, vitality, light, expansion and the outward appearance as well as the direction above and upwards.

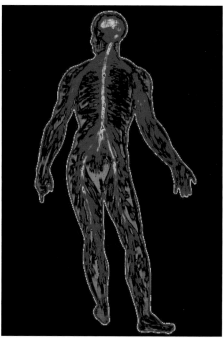

THE RELATIONSHIP BETWEEN YIN AND YANG

Yin and Yang are not absolute, instead they are to be understood in relation to one another. Every object and every living thing, everything in the universe exists of Yin or Yang, but is either more Yin or more Yang depending in what relation it is seen.

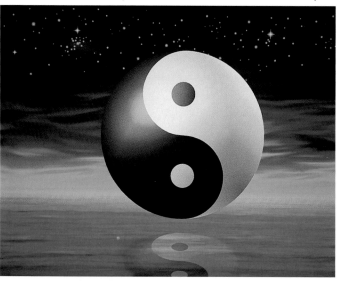

The human body also allows itself to be divided into Yin and Yang: for example the back half of the body is Yang, the front half Yin, the upper half owns more Yang characteristics than the lower half. The outside parts of the body such as skin and hair are more Yang, whereas the inside organs are more Yin. Appropriate characteristics of Yin and Yang can also be divided into Yin and Yang illnesses: illnesses characterised by Yin are connected with weakness, passiveness, cold, and retreat. Counter to that Yang illnesses are portrayed through activity, heat, strength and excitement.

Every Yin or Yang area of any living being, object or state allows itself likewise to be divided into Yin or Yang districts. This process continues – so to speak into infinity. This way you can for instance tell the difference between dark (Yin) and light (Yang). The area "dark" can likewise be divided into very dark (yin) or slightly dark (Yang). The same applies to illnesses, a Yang-illness – characterised by heat and over-activity – can at the same time have Yin-aspects for example weight loss.

son does not only have positive or negative characteristics, but you will find good as well as bad sides to him or her. There is always one rotten apple in the barrel. Every rose has its thorn.

Yin and Yang are in a permanent process of change and balance. Things in which there is more Yin attract Yang and the other way around. If a person is more Yin – then he is more passive and quiet, throughout his life he may become more active, and thereby moves towards being more Yang.

EVERYTHING STRIVES FOR HARMONY

In accordance with the fundamental conviction of eastern philosophy and life vision, all things with regard to Yin and Yang strive for a balance, but nothing can be individual in an ideal balance, because everything is either more Yin or more Yang.

Yin and Yang appear as a dynamic pair of opposites. By combining with the other pole everything is in a balancing out process. This way, things that are more Yin attract Yang and the other way around. You can compare this with the positive and negative poles of a magnet. To understand Yin and Yang you need to start with the realisation that nothing can just be, Yin or Yang. In all things – or inanimate – the existence of both Yin and Yang can simultaneously be found. Only together can they submit a whole. This way a per-

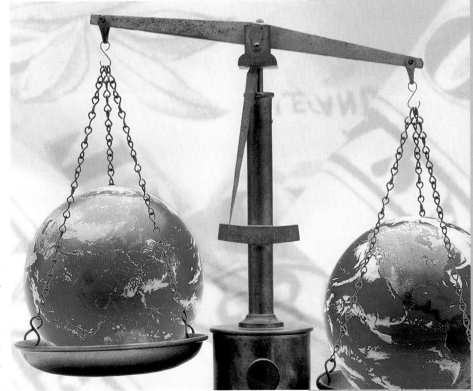

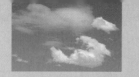

THE FIVE FUNDAMENTAL SUBSTANCES OF THE HUMAN BODY

In traditional Chinese medicine we understand the five fundamental substances as the fundamental Yin and Yang substances of the human body and their relationship to one another. In contrast to western medicine, in which the scientific

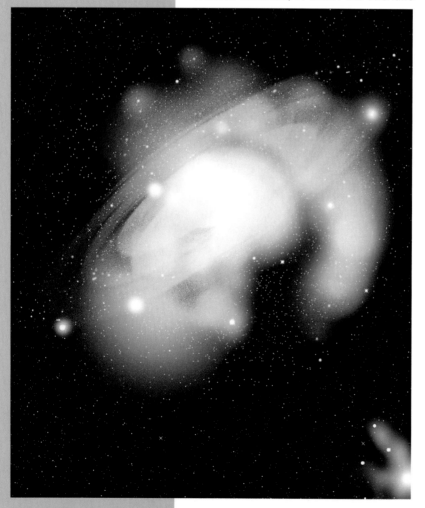

basis – chemistry, biochemistry, anatomy, and physiology – is highly developed, traditional Chinese medicine does not lay nearly as much importance upon these scientific discoveries. In traditional Chinese medicine the cause of illness is not looked for on a cellular basis but is instead determined by the finding of unbalanced energies within the body.

Yin and Yang build the basic concept of Chinese philosophy and therefor also of Chinese medicine. The five fundamental substances Chi, Xue, Jing, Shen, and Jin-Ye refine this basic concept.

CHI

In contrast to the western world, where the attention is focused on matter, energy and vitality play greater roles in the Chinese way of thinking. This opinion also shows itself in traditional Chinese medicine: in the centre you find Chi-energy, which flows throughout the universe binding everything living or inanimate with one another. Western terminology does not have a word with the same meaning as this term. We often find Chi translated as atmosphere, mood, energy, life-energy, vitality or mind.

Chi flows in human bodies, animals, plants, but also in buildings. It flows outwards but reaches into the human body. Every human, every animal, every plant, and every building has its own, personal Chi, which permanently mixes with the Chi from its surroundings. That way everyone is not only connected with their direct surroundings but with the whole universe.

The river of Chi, which flows within us, as well as out of us, decides our moods, our emotions and with this also our psychological and physical constitution.

NORMAL CHI (ZHENG-CHI)

The normal Chi portrays the whole chi of the body. It is generated from three sources:

1. The Original Chi (Yuan-Chi): The original Chi is given to a child by its parents in conception and defines at least a large part of the physical constitution. The original Chi energy is stored in the kidneys.

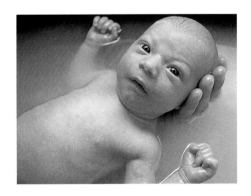

2. The Nutrition Chi (Gu-Chi):

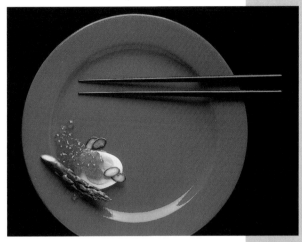

The nutrition Chi comes from the food we take in and digest.

3. The Natural Air Chi (Gong-Chi):

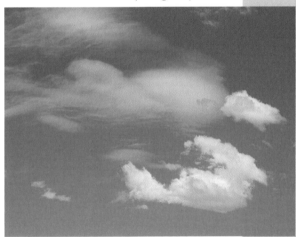

We take this Chi from the air we breathe.

The Normal-Chi is made up of these three chi types. It carries out the following five functions in the body:

1. The source of movement in the body: Included in this are all conscious actions such as walking, running, eating, all automatic muscle movements such as breathing, heartbeat, but also mental activities such as thinking, dreaming etc.

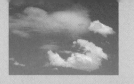

The Chi in the human body is fed by breath and food and supplies various organs with life tonic (Yin) and vitality (Yang). If an organ has a balanced Chi then it functions optimally and is healthy. A possible Chi weakness is normally the result of imbalanced Yin and Yang strengths, this causes the organ to over or under function.

The complete bodily and mental development, such as growth depends upon Chi.

2. Protection of the Body: Chi stops unhealthy influences of the environment from entering the body.

3. The Conversion of Food:
Chi makes sure that the food we consume is converted into other substances such as blood, sweat and urine.

4. Order in the Body:
Chi regulates the secretion of various bodily fluids and is therefore responsible for the organs not shifting and makes sure that blood does not leak out of the vessels.

5. Temperature regulation:
The warming function of Chi takes care of the correct body temperature.

In traditional Chinese medicine the most important types of Chi are:

- Organ-Chi: The organ-Chi decides over the most important organ functions, its activity is defined by the appropriate organ.

- Leading path-Chi: With leading paths you indicate channels and paths through which the Chi can flow.

- Nutrition-Chi: This Chi moves with the blood. It converts the "healthy" contents of the food into blood.

- Defence-Chi: This Chi stops damaging influences from entering the body.

- Breathing-Chi: This Chi is found in the chest area and controls the breathing and heartbeat.

Chi can be disrupted by many influences. When this happens you get a lack of Chi, a broken down Chi, a stagnated Chi or a counter-Chi.

XUE (BLOOD)

The Chinese word Xue does not exactly correspond to the western word blood. In Chinese medicine, because the function of the blood is more important than the localisation of the organs in the body, it is not exactly defined where and through which channels the blood moves. It is important however that the blood, a Yin-substance, permanently circulates the body, feeding it and keeping it,

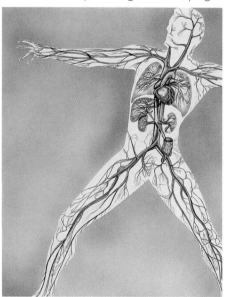

as well as connecting different parts of the body together.

As mentioned before, blood is formed through the conversion of food: the spleen filters a cleansed concentrate out of the

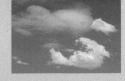

food, this is then transported by the spleen-Chi to the lungs. On its way it is converted into blood by the nutrition-Chi (see page 12). Once inside the lung it is mixed with clean air. There is an interchangeable dependence between Chi and blood, they are inseparably connected to one another. This way Chi creates and moves blood, whereas blood feeds the organs that are responsible for producing Chi. This interchangeable relationship explains the principle of Yin (blood) and Yang (Chi) very well.

It is possible for blood to become imbalanced the same as with chi energy, this leads to blood deficiency or blocked blood. If an organ or the whole body does not receive enough blood, which would mean not enough nutrition, it can be recognised by symptoms such as pale or dry skin, and also in a lack of confidence or a reduced capability to show efficiency. Blocked blood originates from a blockage that stops the blood from flowing harmoniously. A condition like this often shows itself through cysts, tumours, and swollen organs – mainly in the liver.

JING

In traditional Chinese medicine all organic life is based on a substance they call Jing. The body creates the strength to organically change itself with Jing. Jing is depicted as a substance similar to liquid and is the foundation for reproduction and development. How and how fast an organism develops from conception through to death depends upon the change of the Jing. If the Jing finds itself imbalanced you get a Jing deficiency, this

can lead to sexual problems, infertility and premature ageing. Even if these illnesses are congenital, traditional Chinese medi-

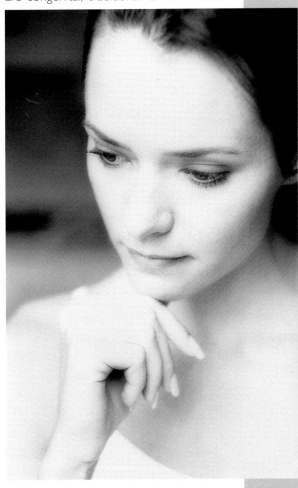

cine associates them with a Jing functional disorder.

As with Xue and Chi, Jing and Chi also depend upon each other, where Jing depicts a Yin and Chi a Yang manifestation.

SHEN

Shen is the only fundamental substance that belongs to a person alone. It embodies the human consciousness. We may thank Shen for our ability to think and make decisions etc. Shen is received during conception from the parents and continues to develop after birth. Opposite to our word "spirit", Shen has a material character. In traditional Chinese medicine Shen only plays a part when in connection with the organism and is as important to the body as the organs. From this basic understanding of Shen we can see that in traditional Chinese medicine there is no separation between body and spirit. Instead Body and spirit are inseparably together. It

is again possible, the same as with the other fundamental substances, that it can become unbalanced. This is noticeable by forgetfulness or worse, in irrationality.

JIN-YE (BODY FLUIDS)

The fifth fundamental substance consists of all body fluids other than blood: sweat, saliva, gastric acids and urine. The Chinese word Jin means clear and light liquid, Ye stands for thick liquid. Body fluids serve to feed skin, hair, flesh, muscles, organs etc. In comparison to the other four fundamental substances, it is obvious that body fluids have less importance.

Body fluids are taken from the food we eat, the Chi from the kidneys absorbs the fluids and controls them. A body fluid deficiency or an imbalance in the body fluids is noticeable through dry skin and dried out mucus membranes. There is also a dependency between fluids and Chi. The fluids are dependent upon Chi as it absorbs the liquid. Chi on the other hand can only stay in balance if the organs, that regulate the Chi, are connected and fed by the bodily fluids.

As fluids are in constant movement, they belong to the Yin-substances.

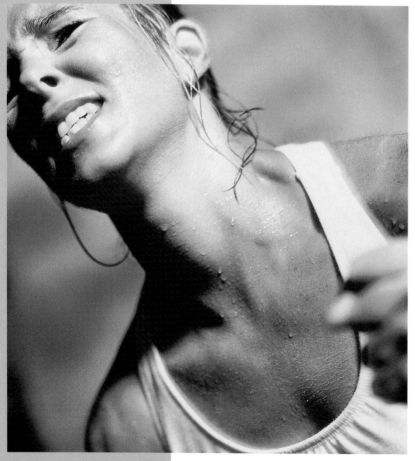

THE FIVE CHANGING PHASES

Essentially the Chinese put all relationships between all types of phenomenon into the categories of Yin and Yang. In ancient China they also used yet another system for categorising phenomenon: the system of the five changing phases, where wood, fire, earth, metal and water are the symbols used to describe all occurrences in the universe. The theory of the five changing phases influences almost the whole traditional Chinese way of thinking and therefore also Chinese medicine. According to eastern philosophy, the interaction of the five changing phases or the five elements earth, wood, fire, metal, and water controls the natural course of phenomenon. It is important to note that these elements are not real, existing substances but instead are symbols and abstract strengths or powers for certain fundamental characters of the matter. Understood this way the five elements improve the principle of Yin and Yang.

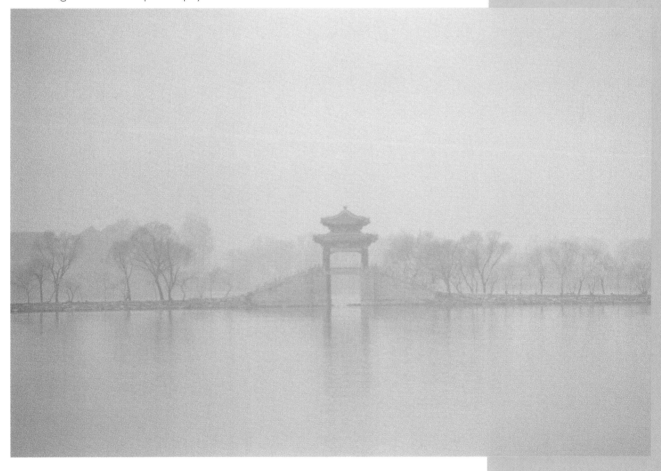

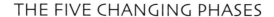

In the cycle of creation, wood feeds the fire when burning, this creates ash. The ash becomes new earth, which allows metals to originate. These draw the morning dew to them – water – which likewise feeds the plants – the wood.

THE RELATIONSHIPS BETWEEN THE FIVE CHANGING PHASES

The relationships between the five changing phases are characterised by two energy flows: There is the circulation of production and the checking cycle. In the creation or production cycle the energy always comes from something else. All the five energies or elements are mothers to their following energy, which is regarded as their child. In the production or creation cycle the energy – Chi – moves clockwise from one element to the next. Every energy brings out the next one, but is weakened by this bringing out, this means every element is exhausted by the next.

Water brings out wood, but is also exhausted by it.

Wood brings out fire, but is in return exhausted by it.

Fire brings out earth, but is also exhausted by it.

Earth brings out metal, but is also exhausted by it.

Metal brings out water, but is also exhausted by it.

The cycle closes.

The checking cycle on the other hand runs in straight lines, always missing the next element. This way the energy kicks in when the next following element is weak. In the following overview the relationships between the five elements is shown again here.

🐚 Water
creates wood, checks fire (when wood is weak), exhausts metal

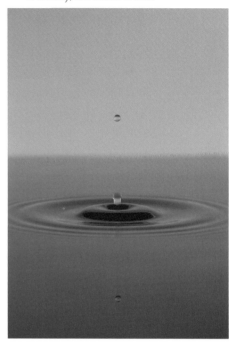

🐚 Wood
creates fire, checks earth (when fire is weak), exhausts water

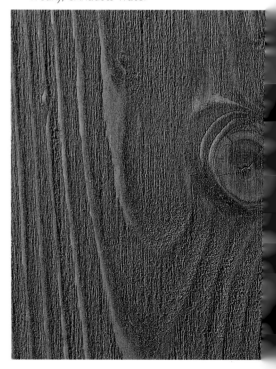

❧ Fire
creates earth, checks metal (when earth is weak), exhausts wood

❧ Metal
creates water, checks wood (when water is weak), exhausts earth

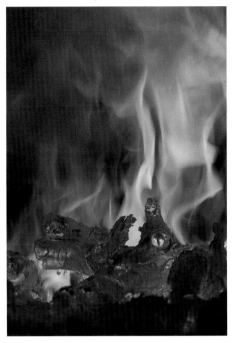

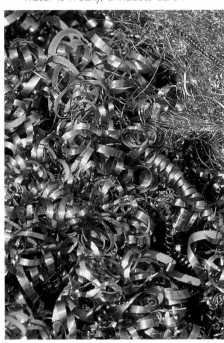

❧ Earth
creates metal, checks water (when metal is weak), exhausts fire

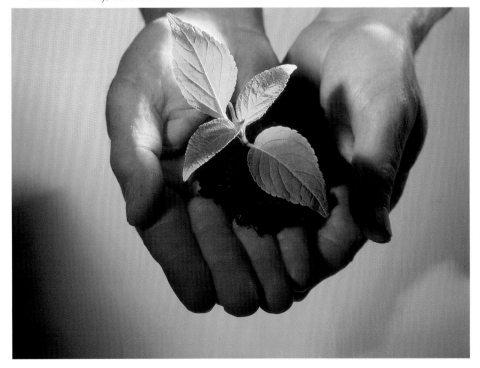

In Chinese philosophy the checking cycle checks the elements. Wood checks earth, when the plants dig through the soil. Earth checks water by absorbing it. Water checks fire by putting it out. Fire checks metal as the heat can melt it. Lastly metal checks wood as the axe chops down the tree.

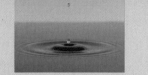

THE IMPORTANCE OF THE FIVE CHANGING PHASES FOR THE HUMAN BODY

It is also possible to perceive the five changing phases in human nature. Although sometimes the transitions in the cycles are so slow that we believe them to be static. Still it is true that everything in nature goes through changes from construction to destruction, so illness can only be a station in an enduring process.

Above all of the Yin- and Yang-organs (heart – small intestines, spleen – stomach, lungs – large intestines, kidneys – bladder, liver – gall bladder, pericardium – triple-warmer) there is one of the five changing phases, which you can see in the chart below. What consequences a weakness in one of the changing phases could have, is explained here in an example: if the metal energy in the lungs is weakened, then not enough or no water energy is created. This reduces the function of the bladder. Symptoms for example would be thirst and strongly concentrated urine. Western medicine would at this point, attempt to normalise the bladder function. Chinese medicine on the other hand fights the illness at the root, which in this case would be in the lungs, with the appropriate herbs. When the metal energy in the lungs is tamed back to normal, it can produce enough water energy for the bladder again.

The five changing phases and their manifestation

	wood	fire	earth	metal	water
Yin-organs	liver	heart pericardium (see page 21)	spleen	lungs	kidneys
Yang-organs	gall bladder	small intestines triple-warmer (see page 24)	stomach	large intestine	bladder
flavour	sour	bitter	sweet	spicy	salty
climate	windy	hot	damp	dry	cold
tissue	tendons	blood vessels	flesh	skin	bones

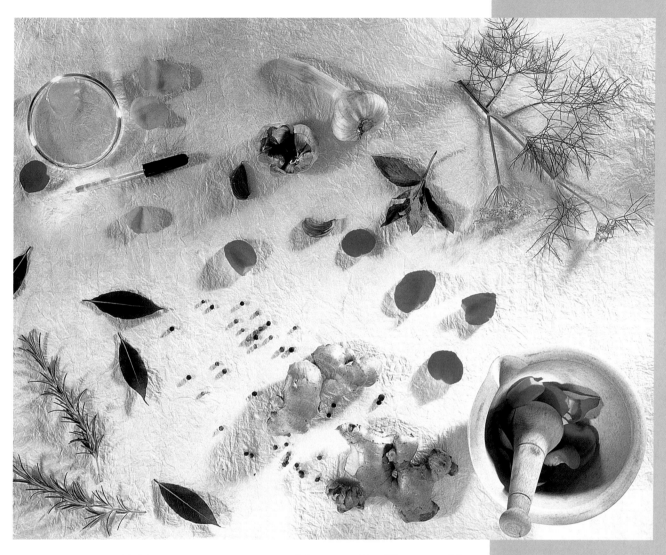

THE FLAVOURS OF THE FIVE CHANGING PHASES

The five changing phases are also related to different flavours, as you will also find again with herbs (see page 39 ff.) and food (see page 32). With this approach metal has a spicy flavour and checks the lungs and the intestines. Herbs and foods with a spicy flavour therefore also have a connection with the lungs and intestines. Most herbs do not just give us one flavour, but provide us with a wide range of flavours with different qualities and form an affinity to many organs. This plays a big part in the mixing of herbs in different remedies, as here the herbs integrate with the organs in a complex way. This explains why Chinese medicine relies on experience, it is only possible to know which mixture will work positively with which illness if you have a broad base of experience in Chinese medicine.

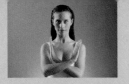
SICKNESS AND HEALTH

THE TWELVE VITAL ORGANS OF THE BODY

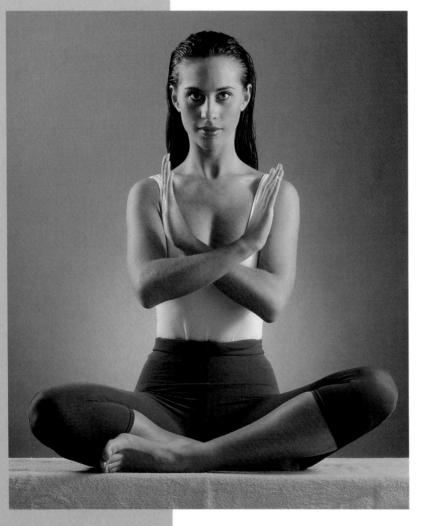

According to the idea of traditional Chinese medicine it is a prerequisite for your health, that the twelve vital organs are all in balance with one another and work in harmony with the fundamental substances. This way the body functions, essential for a healthy being, remain preserved. This means that energy is stored and spread, preserved and transformed, received and eliminated as well as organs being stimulated and calmed. If an even balance is mastered in this area, the person is healthy, not just organically but also psychologically. Here we find, like everywhere else in Chinese philosophy, a striving for harmony, which surfaces time and time again.

Unlike western medicine; an automatic system, that fixes definite locations. Positions and functions of all the organs do not exist in traditional Chinese medicine. For this reason the organs are not 100% the same as the organs known to us, (not only in their location but also in their function). This is why in traditional Chinese medicine, we find on the one hand, there are organs which we do not have, for example the triple-warmer (see page 24), and on the other hand, with a Chinese way of perceiving the organs, we are missing organs which in our opinion carry out important functions. The pancreas is a pertinent example of this point.

Naturally, only a brief outline of these twelve vital organs can be given here. A more detailed description would require not only a lot of time and space, but also a more exact knowledge of traditional Chinese medicine and its philosophical influences.

This book should explain the foundation of traditional Chinese medicine and awaken a healthy interest in this medicine,

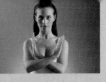

which differs so greatly from our structured learning. Traditional Chinese medicine distinguishes between six Yin-organs heart, pericardium, lungs, spleen, liver and kidneys and six Yang-organs gall bladder, stomach, small intestines, large intestines, bladder and the triple-warmer.

THE SIX
YIN-ORGANS

The task of the Yin-organs is to produce, convert, regulate the flow and store the five fundamental substances of the human (see page 10 ff.). They lie deeper than the Yang organs.

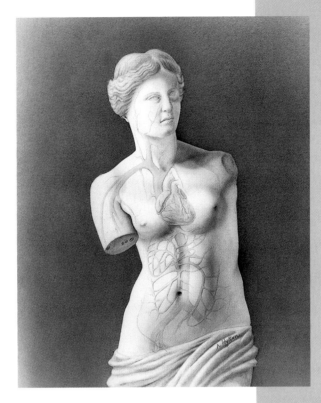

- The Heart

  As the heart (Xin) is more important it determines haemorrhages. This means that the blood flows harmoniously if the heart is healthy. Consequently the heart, veins and blood are all tied closely together. Another task of the heart is to store Shen, the human's consciousness (see page 14). If the heart cannot carry out this task adequately, it manifests itself along with other features in sleeplessness, violent dreams or forgetfulness. It is interesting to note that an unbalanced heart-Chi manifests itself on the tongue. This way a pale tongue indicates a deficiency of blood in the heart and a blue tongue indicates blocked blood in the heart. These conditions can also be recognised in the face: a healthy complexion with a rosy taint shows an adequate supply of blood to the heart, a slightly bluish colouring of the face suggests a blockage of blood in the heart.

- The Pericardium

  Although there is actually little difference between heart and pericardium (Xin-Bao), the pericardium surrounds the heart like an outer protective cover. It is supposed to fend off damaging and straining influences.

- The Lungs

  In traditional Chinese medicine, the lung (Fei) is responsible for breathing. It regulates the complete Chi of the body. Apart from that the lung is involved in the transporting and converting of water in the body.

  With a downward movement, steam condenses and thereby reaches the kidneys, pores and skin. In this way the lung regulates the moisture content of the skin and sweat glands. In this context the lung grants a kind of immune function, as it washes damaging sub-

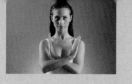

stances out of the body. In addition to this the lung is closely connected with the nose, throat and vocal chords.

🍂 The Spleen

In traditional Chinese medicine the spleen (Pi) is considered the most

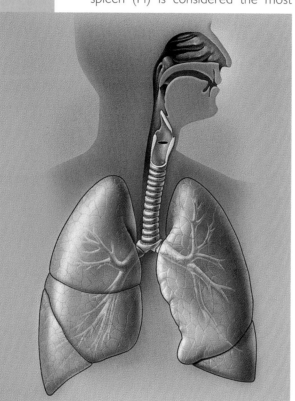

important digestive organ. In the conversion of food to Chi and blood the spleens plays the main part. It is here the components needed to convert food into Chi and blood is withdrawn. In addition to this, the spleen moves the water upwards in the body and is responsible for the blood flowing in the correct paths. Besides this the spleen transports Chi and blood to our muscles; therefore our muscle strength is reliant on the efficiency of the spleens function. The mouth and lips are also closely connected to the spleen.

Only when the spleen-Chi is properly balanced can we tell the difference between the five flavours (see page 19).

🍂 The Liver

The harmonious flowing movement of the five fundamental substances depends on a crucial well-balanced liver-Chi. The liver (Gan) is responsible for supplying all parts of the body with the five fundamental substances. If the liver function becomes impaired, the body's energy will stagnate and will not be able to flow, causing the blood to block. The liver is also partially responsible for a healthy digestion. If the liver-Chi is unbalanced the stomach and spleen can be attacked as the digestion goes in the wrong direction. Besides this the liver controls the secretion of bile, which plays an important part in our digestive system. Lastly the liver regulates our emotions and vice versa, if our emotions are spoilt it has a negative effect on the liver. Liver and emotions therefore find themselves in permanent interaction with one another. A further function of the liver is storing and regulating the blood. It makes sure that during physical activity the body is supplied with adequate blood. When a quiet moment arises, the blood flows back into the liver and is stored there. As a central organ the liver is connected with the eyes and the tendons.

🍂 The Kidneys

The kidneys (Shen) store Jing – a substance that controls reproduction and development (see page 13). As all organs need this substance, all life activ-

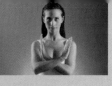

ity is found within the kidneys. In traditional Chinese medicine, premature ageing or ageing of the body without any mental maturity is always traced back to a disharmonious Jing balance in the kidneys. As there is a close connection between the kidneys and the strength and growth of hair and ears, a deterioration of the hair or hearing in old age is traced back to an age determined weakness of the kidney-Jing.

Another task of the kidneys is to maintain the movement and the conversion of the water. As the kidneys store Jing which is responsible for bone marrow production, which in return creates and preserves bone, the kidneys and bones or bone marrow are closely linked.

THE SIX YANG-ORGANS

The task of the Yang-organs is to take the components out of the food, which are used for creating the fundamental substances, and break them down. Then they transport the unwanted matter out of the body. In comparison to the Yin-organs the Yang-organs clearly have a weaker connection to the five fundamental substances.

- The Gallbladder
  The gallbladder (Dan) stores and isolates the bile – a bitter, yellow liquid that is always formed from surplus liver-Chi.
  If and when the need arises, the gallbladder sends the bile down into the stomach, where it becomes part of the digestive process. The liver and the gallbladder are dependent on each

other. An imbalance in the liver impairs the gallbladder and vice versa.

- The Stomach
  In the stomach (Wei) eaten food is digested. So this is where the digestive process begins. From the stomach certain food components are sent to the spleen to be converted into Chi and Xue. Other food components are passed on to the small intestines where they are further digested.

- The Small Intestines
  In the small intestines (Xiao-Chang) the food is broken down again and then passed on to the spleen or the large intestines. Another part is carried straight into the kidneys and bladder.

- The Large Intestines
  The large intestines (Da Chang)

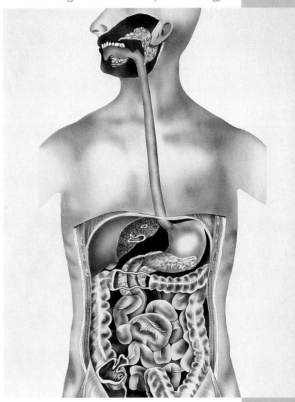

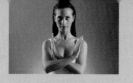

extract the water from the food components that arrive there, the rest is excreted.

🔊 **The Bladder**
The bladder (Pang-Guang) expels the urine that arrives there from the kidneys. It is formed from the components that flow into the kidneys, from out of the lungs and small and large intestines.

🔊 **The Triple-Warmer**
Even in classical Chinese literature you will find many different statements concerning this organ, which according to the opinion of many Chinese doctors only has one name, but cannot be located. It virtually creates the link between the organs that deal with water regulation, mainly kidneys, lungs and spleen as well as small intestines and bladder. It can be equated to our metabolism.

THE UNUSUAL ORGANS

Apart from the six Yin- and Yang-organs traditional Chinese medicine also recognises the six unusual organs, which are brain, bone, marrow, veins, womb and gallbladder. The gallbladder also belongs to the Yang-organs.

THE SEVEN EMOTIONS (QI-QING)

In contrast to western medicine Chinese medicine does not recognise any separation between body and spirit. Conse-

quently it is no wonder that the Chinese include the emotional life when diagnosing an illness.

We know from Chinese understanding of the seven emotions, which are still considered exceptionally important today when diagnosing.

They are joy, irritability, sorrow, melancholia, fear and dread. The difference between sorrow and melancholia or fear and dread is not only difficult for us to distinguish, but can only be gradually understood in Chinese medicine.

If all the seven emotions are in balance there is harmony. If one of the emotions gets out of hand for a long period of time or suddenly a serious imbalance takes place, the Chi has an effect on the other fundamental substances and can cause illness.

As the seven emotions are closely linked to the organs (see marginal comment) an imbalance of the Chi in these organs can put the body and spirit out of balance. The reverse also applies.

The seven emotions or their imbalance are not to be considered as the only cause of illness. Only together with other factors such as the five fundamental substances or the twelve vital organs do they form a foundation for sickness and health.

THE SIX EVILS (LIU-YIN)

You will find the term the six evils in Chinese medical encyclopaedias in the following context: When the six environmental energies wind, cold, heat, dampness, dryness and fire become too strong or appear outside of their corre-

Traditional Chinese medicine values the spirit and body of a person as a single unit. This way every emotion is directly linked to an organ and its functional environment: Joy is linked to the heart and circulation, irritability is linked to the liver and metabolism, sorrow is linked to the breathing functions, melancholia or worry are linked to the spleen and digestive system, fear and dread are linked with the kidneys and urogenital functions.

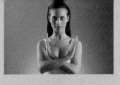

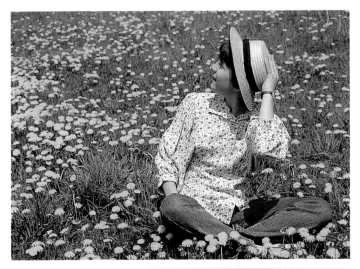

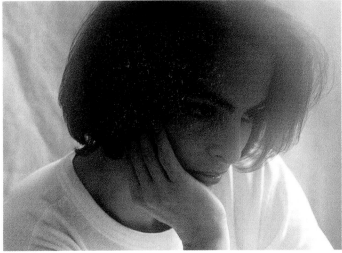

An excess of an emotion has an enduring influence on the psyche and brings about a certain posture, which in the long run can cause pain especially with certain movements. This way excessive joy causes exaggerated and fast body movements (psyche: nervous, hysterical). Melancholia or worry cause a heavy unsupported head (psyche: pondering, melancholy). Sorrow leads to a rounded back and a weakened body (psyche: shy). Fear and dread lead to tense back muscles (psyche: tired, easily shocked, tense). Irritability causes body tension, and a loud voice (psyche: excited, rage).

sponding season, then they become a cause of illness, and they are called the six evils. Once again we see that harmony, balance and equilibrium decide over the single factors – in this case, the environmental-energies.

In traditional Chinese medicine the six evils are summarised as the "outside causes of illness". In contrast to the seven emotions which form the "inner cause of illness" (see page 24) the six evils can, if they become more strongly pronounced, imbalance the Chi and thereby weaken the immune system, which can no longer fight back the negative influences of the environment.

The six evils correspond with the understanding of ancient Chinese medicine as climatic situations, which are, wind, cold, heat, dampness, dryness and fire. Apart from these weather conditions, today we have other factors as well for example air-conditioning, heating, pollution etc. These can gravely influence our Chi more negatively that the six evils.

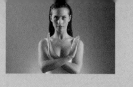

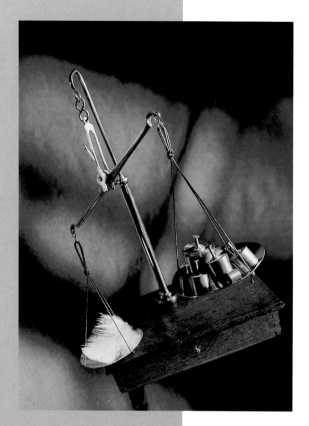

WIND

The Chines associate wind (Feng) with movement, which it produces where otherwise it would be still. This means wind arouses change, disturbs the energy out of its even flow. Wind is consequently a Yang element. As an evil wind rarely occurs alone, instead it occurs mainly in connection with heat or cold.

In traditional Chinese medicine it is assumed that the "malicious" wind mainly moves upwards and outwards. It is manifested in the face, skin, sweat glands and

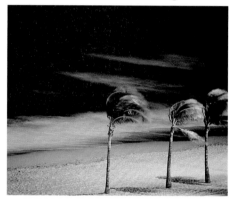

lungs. The characteristic manifestations of the evil wind are fever, draught sensitivity, headaches, an abrupt manner, closed respiratory passages and a sore throat.

COLD

In contrast to wind, cold (Han) belongs to the Yin-elements. The Chinese associate cold with winter. If the immune system is weakened then a person is more sensitive to cold, the circulation does not function adequately, cold shivers, fever, and even physical pain can occur.

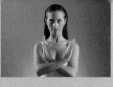

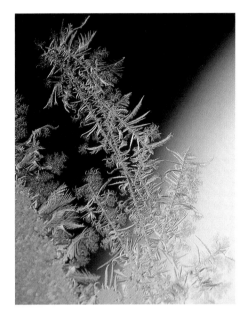

Just think about how for example cold hands can hurt. The effect of outside cold is increased when inner cold already exists. Inner cold is caused by a lack of Yang in the vital organs.

HEAT

The evil heat (Re) belongs on the other hand to the Yang-elements. The illnesses caused by this evil are noticed the most during summer when heat is at its strongest. If someone is exposed to too much heat then over perspiring, fever, red face, strong headaches could occur. In this case cold is sought and heat is avoided.

DAMPNESS

Dampness (Shi) belongs to late summer and is a Yin-element. Dampness is connected to the attribute "heavy". An excessive amount of dampness can lead to cold sweats, stiff and painful joints as well as tiredness and lethargy.

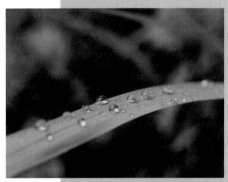

DRYNESS

Too little humidity, dryness (Zao) is connected with autumn in China. Dryness has a negative influence on the function of the lungs. In connection with other evils such as heat, cold or wind, dryness can cause various illnesses in the respiratory tract. With a connection between lung (Yin) and intestines (Yang), constipation can also be traced back to dryness.

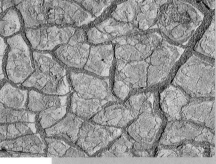

FIRE

In traditional Chinese medicine fire is seen as too much of one of the environmental energies or as a meeting of lots of strongly developed environmental-energies.

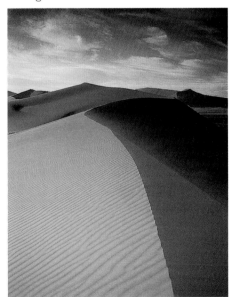

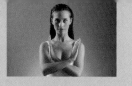

THE WAY OF LIFE

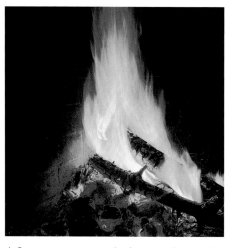

A fire can permanently damage the twelve vital organs. An example: a respiratory tract illness caused by the evil dryness could degenerate into lung emphysema (swelling of the lung) or even into lung cancer if the evil dryness is not avoided soon enough.

In Chinese culture the correct way of life is considerably important to whether a person is healthy or ill. The first desired value here is a life, which is in harmony with the environment, yes the whole universe: this means that between Yin and Yang and the single emotions there is a harmonious balance.

The way of life is determined by three factors, they are correct diet (see next chapter), the right amount of sexual activity, which of course cannot be defined, but instead depends upon society and social circumstances, and physical activity at the right time. The latter should, according to Chinese standards, always be in harmony with the universe, the season, the condition of the body and of course also with age. So it is also important here to take Yin and Yang into consideration.

This means Ying-times (youth, spring, morning) are pronounced through activity and the Yin-times (old age, winter, evening) through peacefulness. Even in Yang-times you should check the correct amount of physical movement, because too much could lead through the spleen to a lack of Chi and Xue.

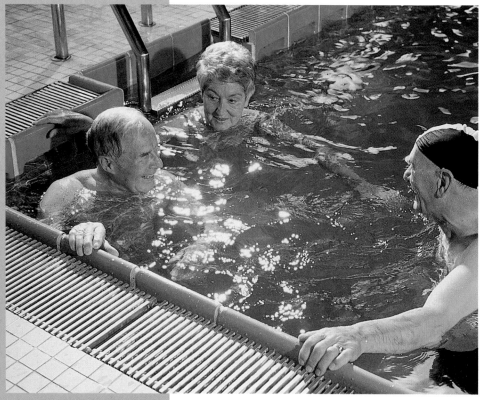

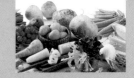

THE SIGNIFICANCE OF THE CORRECT DIET IN TRADITIONAL CHINESE MEDICINE

There is a saying often used in China, "Food is medicine, medicine is food." This explains the valued place a healthy balanced diet has in Chinese medicine. Even in western medicine the health advantages of a balanced diet is becoming more and more recognised. Today a healthy diet also plays an important part in our lives.

The Chinese still treat a lot of small health problems with a meal, in which they include appropriate ingredients specially for healing health problems. Food has different properties, according to the Chinese way of thinking. They influence our body- and organ-Chi in various ways. Of course you should not forget that Chinese medicine cannot heal serious illnesses by only keeping to a certain diet. But a har-monious diet orientated to the characteristics of the food, prevents illness and supports in view an intact health.

A balanced diet in accordance with ancient Chinese herbal medicine is put together from various components. The following will explain how taking notice of a few important rules on nutrition will make a change towards a healthy body and an intact immune system.

According to Chinese herbal medicine food and life, and nutrition and medicine are equal, because all living things do not live on oxygen and water alone, but also on food. All food is a medicine, which gradually through the years and centuries decides over health and illness.

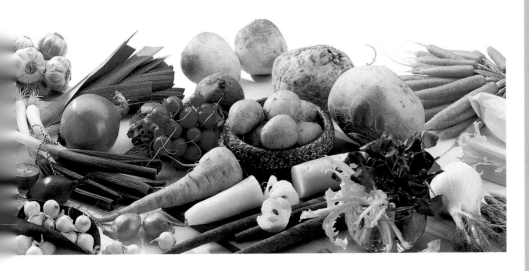

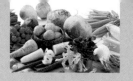

To explain the classifications "hot" or "warm" and "cool" or "cold" temperaments of food, here are two examples: The zucchini has a cool temperament even when heated up. On the other hand cherries have a warm temperament even when eaten straight from the fridge.

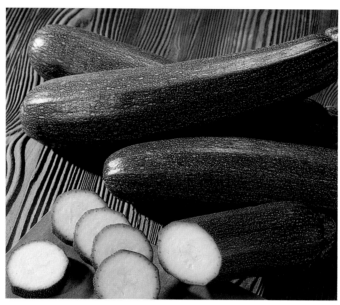

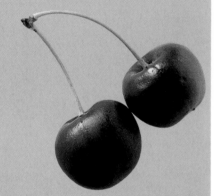

THE EFFECTS OF NUTRITION

YIN- AND YANG-FOODS – THE TWO TEMPERAMENTS

As throughout all Chinese medicine, the focus of attention in diet is on harmony and balance. Chinese medicine distinguishes food and medicinal plants by two fundamental units; cool or cold and warm or hot. This is not meant as the physical temperature of the food, but as the effect it has on the body. The classifications found on the following pages are not the result of an arbitrary mood, but are the result from centuries of experience and study that traditional Chinese medicine has gained.

Hot and warm foods belong to the Yang-elements, they have a hot or warm temperament. For medical reasons they should especially be taken when the inner cold is strong.

Element	Fire	Earth	Metal	Water	Wood
Flavour	bitter	sweet	spicy	salty	sour
Scent	burnt	fragrant	sharp	foul	rancid
Area of effect	heart	spleen	lung	kidney	liver
Effect	cleanses, cools	strenthens, harmonises	divides, uplifts	dissolves, carries away	draws together, seals

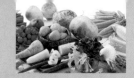

This is why it is appropriate to eat more meat on cold days. Meat can, as a warming energy-tonic, (for example in the form of a strengthening soup prepared with medicinal herbs) fight against a slight freezing constitution that is called a Yang-weakness. In reverse to this fresh fruit (apples, pears) and vegetables are known as cool or cold foods.

THE FIVE FLAVOURS

Foods, the same as medicinal herbs, are categorised into five flavours and the five appropriate elements (see chart on page 30). Depending on the flavour, foods display different effects. The same applies to the scent that food exudes. They are categorised into five elements and their appropriate organ.

THE DIRECTION EFFECT OF FOOD

Food does not only have flavour, scent and a temperament, but also a directional effect on the body: Some foods "lift" the organs and body-Chi, others "lower" it. It is also possible that a food does not influence the body at all and is thereby neutral. This condition is known as hovering.
If the aim is to lower the energy in the body, for example to reduce the amount of energy in the head to relieve headaches, then you should eat food which contains a lowering direction effect. This is of course a simple explanation. In reality the

connections are more complicated, yet it is still possible to positively affect the body and spirit by keeping to a few important rules. The chart on the next page shows a

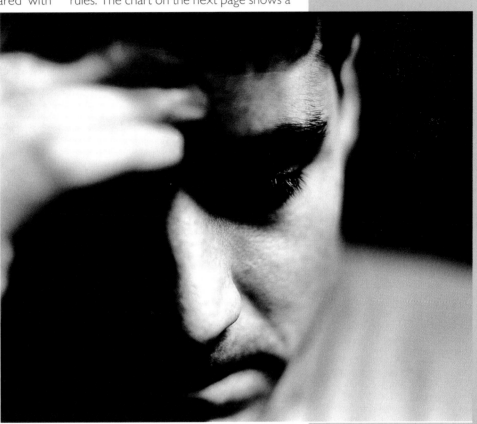

few chosen foods, which are also known in Europe, and the characteristics they have.

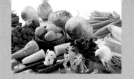

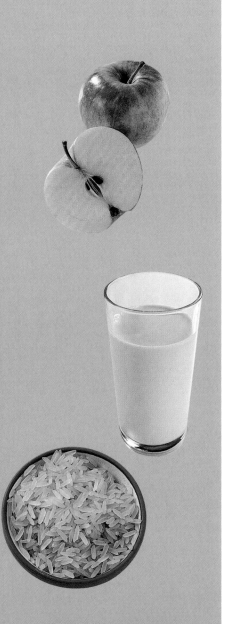

Food	Flavour	Temperament	Direction effect
Apple	sweet, sour	cool	lowering
Asparagus	spicy, bitter	warm	hovering
Beef	sweet, salty	warm	lowering
Carrots	sweet	warm	lifting
Cauliflower	spicy, sweet	neutral	lowering
Chicken egg	sweet	neutral	lifting
Chicken	sweet	warm	lifting
Cod	salty, sweet	neutral	lowering
Duck	sweet, salty	neutral	hovering
Endives	bitter	cold	lowering
Garlic	spicy	hot	lifting
Goose	sweet	neutral	hovering
Honey	sweet	warm	lifting
Lentils	sweet	neutral	lowering
Maize	sweet	warm	lifting
Milk	sweet	neutral	lifting
Onions	spicy, sweet	warm	lifting
Pears	sweet	cool	lifting
Pork	sweet, salty	neutral	lowering
Potato	sweet	neutral	hovering
Rice	sweet	warm	lifting
Salmon	salty	cool	lowering
Salt	salty	cool	lowering
Wheat	sweet	cool	lowering

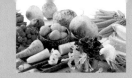

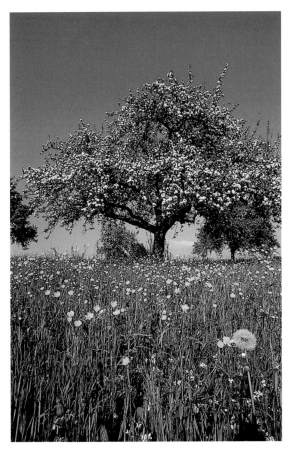

ADAPTING YOUR DIET
TO SUIT THE SEASON

In Chinese medicine the way of eating is strongly dictated by the five elements and with them the five seasons: spring, summer, late summer, autumn and winter.

In spring, when energy needs to get "out" again you should eat food that lifts and strengthens the body-Chi. These desired effects are obtainable in food with the flavour "spicy". The season should also be considered, in spring everything opens up so sprouts and young vegetables are important.

In the summer when the outside heat is at its strongest, foods with the following characteristics are recommended: sour, cool, but not cooling and light. In late summer you should favour harmonising foods. These are mainly meals, which are in keeping with the important rules listed at the side of this page.

In autumn it is recommended to eat foods, which will moisten, this is to help stimulate the production of the body fluids.

In winter the Yang-energy also the warm-energy needs to be preserved. All foods with a warm or hot temperament are suitable for this season.

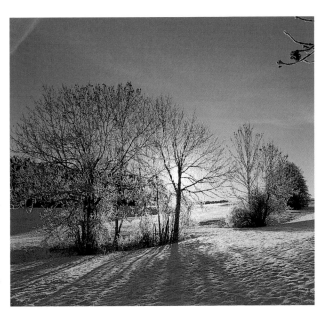

A Few
Important Rules

- *Eat one bread meal and two hot meals every day*

- *Use rice instead of potatoes*

- *Replace coffee with green tea*

- *Only drink wine and beer in small doses*

- *Refrain from drinking high percentage alcohol*

- *Drink plenty of mineral water*

- *Do not mercilessly over boil vegetables, steam them for a short time only, so they still taste crisp, cut them up small while preparing*

- *Pay attention to quality when food shopping*

- *Only use foods appropriate to their season, so no strawberries and peaches in winter*

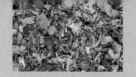

CHINESE
MEDICINAL HERBS

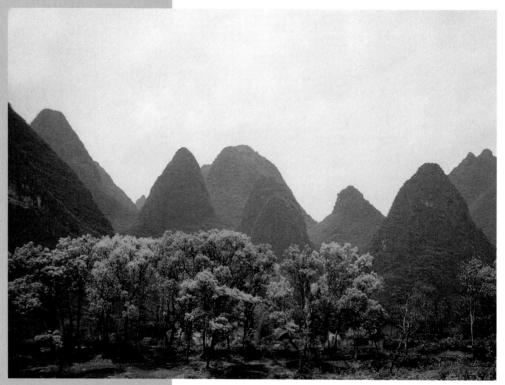

In traditional Chinese medicine, herbal medicine, being the oldest branch of this science, plays an important if not the most important roll. According to legend the emperor Shen Nung is to thank for discovering herbal medicine 5000 years ago. In the 16th century doctor and nature researcher Li Shizhen wrote his famous outline of herbal medicine, which is made up of 52 scrolls. In these scrolls there are 1,892 medicine and over 10,000 remedies (compare with page 6).

The origin of herbal medicine was taken from the mountains of ancient China. There, Taoist hermits searched for the secret elixir of life, which was supposed to make humans immortal. Only after many

hundreds of years did the Taoists realise that this elixir exists in a spiritual form and has to come from the human itself. In their long search they discovered that many herbs have a healing quality and when used in the correct dosage and mixture can be very useful for humans. This shows how herbal medicine was a "waste product" of the search for the elixir and immortality.

In traditional Chinese medicine the centre of focus is not the treatment of an illness, but the treatment of the patient by helping to correct the imbalance of the energies. All the herbs used in traditional Chinese medicine have a natural affinity to a certain organ and the appropriate energy. This is how medicinal herbs can rebalance the energy to their ideal status. Today traditional Chinese medicine recognises around 2,000 medicinal plants, but only around 300 of them are used.

Out of this extensive chemist of medicinal herbs. The herbs listed in this book later have been selected from this extensive natural chemist of medical herbs as herbs known to us. Following this selection of herbs you will find a couple of still classical remedies from traditional Chinese medi-

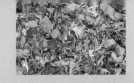

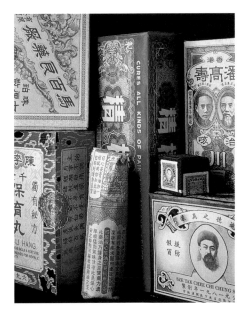

cine. Again here the ingredients consist only of plants, which you can easily obtain through your chemist.

PREPARATION OF THE HERBS

In traditional herbal medicine herbs are boiled (see below) and served as a brew or tea before meals throughout the day. The dry powder formed medicine on the other hand is not boiled, but taken mixed with water. In this next section we will show you various types of herb preparations for healing purposes. The appropriate amounts are found in the herb guide starting on page 39.

BREW (DEKOKT, TANG)

The oldest method of preparing medicinal herbs is a brew. When making a brew all the vital elements of the herb seep into the stock. Like this it can be easily absorbed by the body.

Directions:

- Weigh the herbs
- Put the herbs into a glass or ceramic pan (never use metal when preparing herbs)
- Add 3 to 4 cups of water
- Bring the mixture to the boil
- Simmer at a low temperature with a closed lid until about 1/2 or 1/3 of the liquid is boiled down
- using a piece of muslin placed in a sieve separate the liquid and the herbs
- put the liquid to one side
- boil the herbs again with 2 cups of water until 1/3 or 1/2 of the water has evaporated.

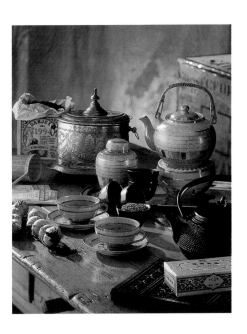

If you ever journey to China or Hong-Kong, you should most definitely visit a Chinese "chemist". The extensiveness of herbs, minerals and animal products kept there is overwhelming. More often now the containers also have English names next to the Chinese. The herbal prescriptions are prepared directly on the counter with the use of hand held scales and an abacus for weighing and arithmetic. Specialised Chinese chemists are still few, but are becoming more and more popular in Britain today (see page 62 for more information).

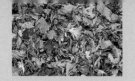

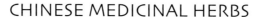

- sieve the liquid together with the first batch, again using a piece of muslin in a sieve
- separate into equal portions for the day and drink throughout the day warm – but not heated in the microwave – drink the brew at intervals during the day

POWDER (SAN)

The herbs can be grounded into a fine powder in a coffee grinder or in a food processor. In contrast to boiling, herbs in a powdered form are not as quickly or as intensively effective, instead the effect lasts longer. The best and easiest way to take herbs in this form is directly on a spoon washed down with warm water or with warm Japanese rice wine (Sake).

Capsules, pastes or pills can be made with powder, but it is not easy and should be left for a chemist to do. Ask for the herbs to be made into a very fine powder and filled into gelatine capsules size 00 (equivalent of about 1g substance).

You can also make an infusion tea from pulverised herbs.

This is how to prepare an infusion tea:

- put the appropriate amount of herbs into a cup
- fill with boiling water
- leave for 3 to 5 minutes
- drink the tea at intervals during the day

PASTE

The production of a paste (Gao) from powder follows these steps:

- put the powdered herbs into a large bowl
- mix with as much honey required to form a thick paste
- take 1 teaspoon as often as required throughout the day and wash down with warm water

OINTMENT (YIO)

Herbal ointments for external use are made up of a mixture of fine herbal powder and a base of beeswax, lanolin or almond oil.

This is how to make an ointment:

- Gently heat the oily base
- Add the powder
- Store in an airtight container (not metal)

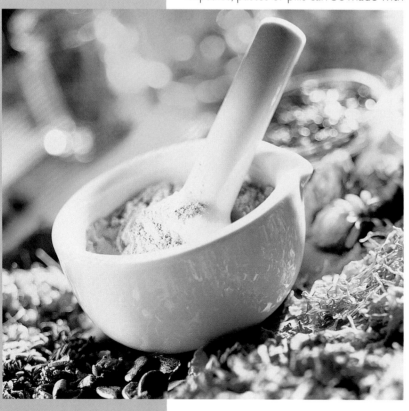

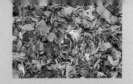

PREPARATION OF THE HERBS

TINCTURE

An effective tincture can be gained by pickling the herbs in a high percentage alcohol (vodka, rum or brandy) for many months. Like with the brew, the vital elements and energies of the herbs are absorbed quickly by the body. Tinctures should be used with plants that have a stimulating effect.

This is how to produce a tincture:

- Put the correct amount of chopped or cut up herbs into a container (not metal) – cover with 6 litres of high per-

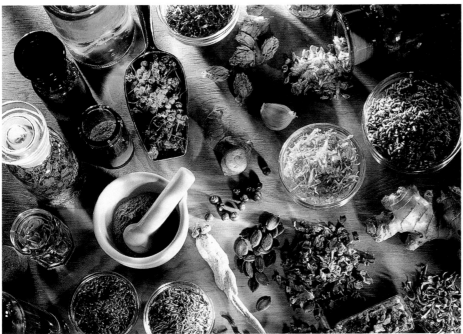

centage alcohol
- Close the lid making sure it is airtight
- Leave for at least 3 months, shake occasionally
- Then pour half the liquid through a fabric filter into a sealable container
- Pour a new 3 litres of alcohol over the herbs and leave for another 3 months

- Lastly drain out the liquid into the container, the herbs are no longer needed

In this way you will acquire around 9 litres of effective herb tincture, which is to be kept in an airtight container. You can add honey or sugar to the tincture if necessary to taste.

Not only plants are used

Traditional Chinese medicine recognises not only the use of plants, but also of minerals and animal products in herbal medicine. There is a lot of controversial discussion, not only in the western world, particularly about the use of animal products for healing purposes. Protection of species is not the only reason you will not find the majority of these healing products with animal origin (tortoise shells, tiger-bones, or bear-gallbladders) here. Using remedies that exclusively contain plant extracts you can also achieve very good successful healing remedies.

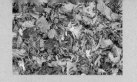

CHARACTERISTICS OF THE HERBS

All Chinese medicines and, therefore, also the herbs, own certain fundamental characteristics and a special temperament behaviour. This is why we have medicinal herbs with:

- "Hot" characteristics: They help when cold and shivering occurs and has a high degree of effect.
- "Warm" characteristics: These are also used when cold and shivering occurs, but do not have such a high degree of effect as herbs with "hot" characteristics. They stimulate the body functions and have an effect on bodily weakness.
- "Cold" characteristics: These are used to treat illnesses accompanied by fever or burning.
- "Cool" characteristics: They have the same effect as herbs with "cold" characteristics, except they are not as distinctive. These medicinal herbs are put into use when someone has a fever or in summer heat.

Herbs with heating, warming characteristics are Yang-herbs. They warm the organism, stimulate the metabolism and the functions of the vital organs. Herbs with cooling, cold characteristics reduce the flow of energies and with that the metabolism and have a calming affect on the vital organs.

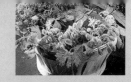

A GUIDE TO CHINESE MEDICINAL HERBS

ALOE

Latin name: Aloe barbadensis

Chinese name: Lu hui

Botany: This stemless, juicy plant can grow up to 15m high, the orange-brown to black leaves are smooth or prickly, the edges of the leaves are toothed.

Found In: Africa, India, Caribbean Islands, the Mediterranean and in some further parts of south east Asia

Used parts of the plant: Pressed juice from fresh leaves is sold in irregular shaped pieces about 2cm in width.

The relevant organs: Liver, stomach, large intestines

Energy: Very cold

Flavour: Very bitter

Effects: According to traditional Chinese medicine, Aloe calms the liver energy and reduces fever and heat. It has a slight laxative effect but can also induce radical bowl movements; it strengthens the stomach functions, regulates menstruation; acts as a germicide and is cooling, supports the regulation of blood pressure by removing deposits from in the vessels.

Areas of application: In traditional medicine aloe is used to fight a lifting liver-fire and too much heat in the large intestines. For internal use; aloe is suitable for chronic constipation and its accompanying skin problems, infected stomach lining, stomach ulcers, poor digestion, stomach ache and indigestion; it is also used for low blood pressure, irregular menstruation cycles, head aches, numbness, complaints because of a liver infection, as well as bowl parasites. Used externally, aloe helps against premature hair loss, burns, sunburn, skin injuries, insect bites, chilblains, athlete's foot, acne and haemorrhoids.

Dosage: The pressed juice should be used internally mixed with water as follows:

for strengthening of the stomach: 0,1–0,2 g

as a mild laxative: 0,3–0,6 g

for a radical bowl movement: 0,8–1,0 g

For external use, rub a little of the freshly pressed juice undiluted onto the effected area.

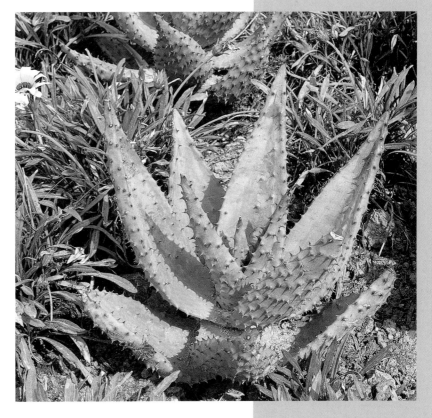

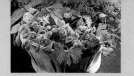

Not to be used in the case of: Children, who have tendencies to empty-cold-symptoms (pale, delicate, prone to colds), constipation, pregnancy or during breast-feeding, adults should not exceed the stated dosages above.

Incompatible with: None

CHINESE WILD PARSNIP (ARCHANGELICA)

Latin Name: Angelica Sinesis

Chinese Name: Dang gui

Botany: An annual, scented plant with brown, fleshy roots, which strongly branch out; highly aromatic plant with a slight bittersweet flavour, which is similar to celery.

Found in: Mainly in middle and west China but also in Japan.

Used parts of the plant: Roots

The relevant organs: Liver and spleen

Energy: Warm

Flavour: Bitter, sweet and slightly spicy.

Effects: According to traditional Chinese medicine, Chinese Wild parsnip tones the blood, it stimulates and regulates menstruation, strengthens the vital organs, eases pain, calms, stimulates the appetite, improves tone of muscle and strengthens the immune system.

Areas of application: According to traditional Chinese, Chinese Wild Parsnip treats empty blood, other areas of application are weak or painful menstruation, pre-menstrual syndrome (PMS), headaches, pain from injuries or operations and loss of appetite.

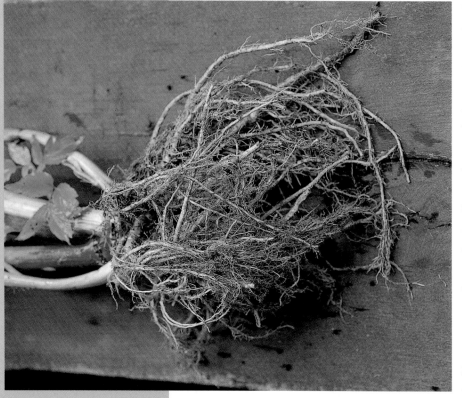

Dosage: For painful irregular menstruation. Brew a whole uncut plant in 2 cups of water. Boil the liquid down to 1 cup and drink half in the morning and half before going to bed on an empty stomach.

Not to be used in the case of: Diarrhoea

Incompatible with: Fresh ginger herbs from the Acorus-family and sea algae

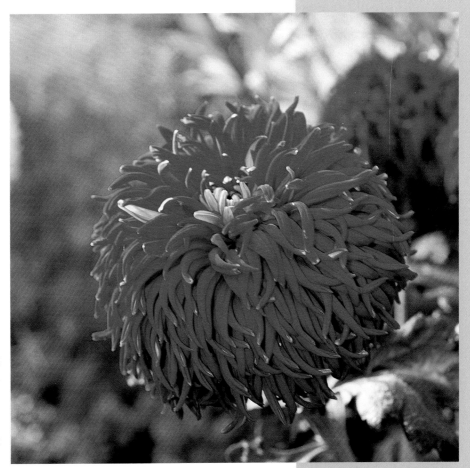

Distinctive features: Angelica is used in western herbal medicine for women's complaints such as irregular menstruation, bleeding during pregnancy, etc.

New studies have found substances similar to oestrogen in the plant. They are called phyto-oestrogen. They are responsible for the menstruation regulating characteristics.

Angelica is the most balanced Yin tonic and forms the companion piece to ginseng, the perfect Yang tonic. A combination of both herbs gives a full and balanced tonic for Yin and Yang energies.

to heal headaches, dizziness, blurred vision (through a defect in the kidneys and liver), raised blood pressure, and numb extremities.

Dosage: For an infusion tea put 8–10g of dried petals into a large teapot (not metal) fill with one litre of boiling water. Pour out after 15–30 minutes drink frequently from the warm or slightly cooled tea throughout the day. The petals can be used up to three times.

CHRYSANTHEMUM

Latin name: Chrysanthemum morifolium

Chinese name: Ju hua

Botany: This plant rarely grows higher than 50cm, it has small flowers in autumn with pink striped yellow petals, pale yellow dried petals with a bitter sweet flavour (illustrated to the right is the red species Indicum-Hybriden)

Found in: Particularly cultivated in China and Japan for medicinal purpose

Used parts of the plant: Petals

The relevant organs: Lungs, liver

Energy: Cool

Flavour: Pleasant, but bitter

Effects: According to traditional Chinese medicine the plant eliminates inner heat and nourishes the blood, it lowers fever and cools, it can lower raised blood pressure and improve vision.

Areas of application: In traditional Chinese medicine it is used against wind and inner heat. It is also used

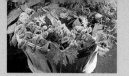

For Chrysanthemum wine cover 20–30 g of petals with 1 litre rice wine (preferably Japenese Sake) or 1 litre sherry, leave for 1–2 weeks to infuse. Drink 25–30 ml 2 or 3 times a day on an empty stomach for poor digestion or circulation as well as nervous complaints.

Distinctive features: Chrysanthemum tea

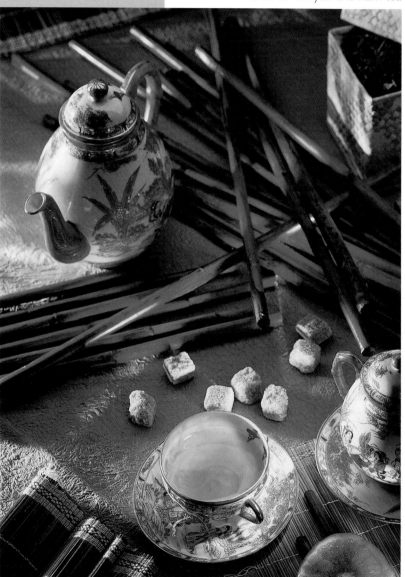

infusions – whether used internally or as a rinse – are a wonderful treatment for swollen, inflammed and itchy eyes.

PURPLE STEM ANGELICA

Latin name: Angelica atropurpurea
Chinese name: Chiang huo
Botany: A species of Angelica villosa; the colour varies from dark purple to green; the roots form wedges from brittle, woody tissue, which has red bark fibres between the inner and outer skin.
Found in: West China
Used parts of the plant: Roots
The relevant organs: Kidneys and bladder
Energy: Warm
Flavour: Spicy and bitter
Effects: According to traditional Chinese medicine, the herb eases inner heat and helps to detoxify the body through the skin; promotes the forming of sweat to relieve water retention through the skin, eases pain and inflammation in rheumatism.
Areas of application: According to traditional Chinese medicine, it is used to treat, inner heat, numbness, blood-shot eyes, loss of speech through a stroke, arthritic and rheumatic pain.
Dosage: Boil 3–6 g and drink in 2 doses on an empty stomach.

GENTIAN

Latin name: Gentiana scabra
Chinese name: Lung dan tsao
Botany: This perennial plant has blue, bell shaped petals and long thin leaves. The roots contain the bitter substances Gentiopicrin, Gentiamarin and Gentin as well as Trisaccharid Gentianose.
Found in: China and Japan and similar species in Europe
Used parts of the plant: Roots
The relevant organs: Liver and gall bladder

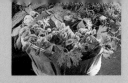

Energy: Very cold

Flavour: Very bitter

Effects: In traditional Chinese medicine, Gentian cools the liver energy, eliminates inner heat, it stops swelling, lowers fever, strengthens the stomach, and eases pain and inflammation in rheumatism.

Areas of application: In traditional Chinese medicine, it is used to treat symptoms of hot humidity, jaundice, diarrhoea caused by too much heat, sore throat, painful and swollen eyes, rheumatic complaints, pustulous abscesses caused by liver poisoning, diabetes, inflammation of the gall bladder and gall stones.

Dosage: Brew 2,5 g and drink in 2 doses after meals. Powder: 2–3 g pure, as a capsule or tea infusion, 2 doses after meals.

Distinctive features: Gentian has been used in western as well as eastern medicine for a long time. It stimulates the digestion and raises circulation in the stomach area. Gentian calms an over-active energy of the spleen and pancreas and can therefore, delay the development of diabetes. It also stops already existing diabetes from progressing further.

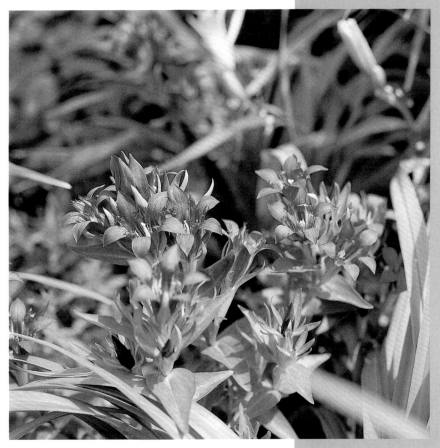

FENNEL

Latin name: Foeniculum vulgare

Chinese name: Hui hsiang

Botany: A perennial, aromatic plant, which grows up to 1–2 metres with small, delicate leaves and yellow petals, grey-brown seeds, and with a similar scent to aniseed. It has 8 mm long, furrowed schizocarp.

Found in: The Middle East, Southern Africa and Southern Europe

Used parts of the plant: The fruits

The relevant organs: Liver, kidneys, spleen and stomach

Energy: Warm

Flavour: Spicy

Effects: In traditional Chinese medicine, Fennel strengthens the stomach energy, warms the kidney energy and has a balancing effect on energy.

Important:

An excessive overdose of Fennel can damage the eyes!

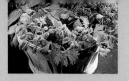

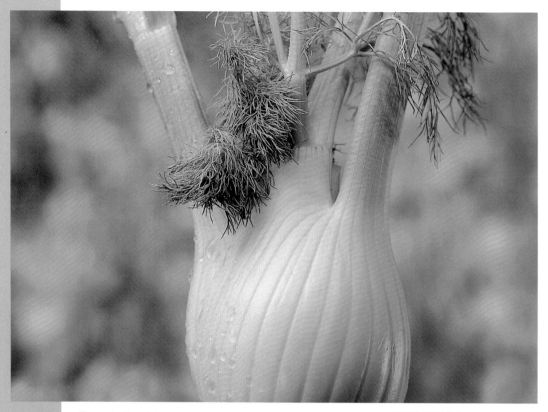

Fennel stimulates, eases coughs, prompts the body to cough up phlegm and stimulates the appetite.

Areas of application: In traditional Chinese medicine, Fennel is used for complaints caused by wind and inner cold, especially in the stomach; for weak digestion, too much stomach acid, cold and pain in the stomach, nausea and vomiting caused by stomach upsets.

Dosage: Brew 3–5 g and drink in 3 doses on an empty stomach. For a powder, roast the Fennel in a dry pan until it gives off a scent then pulverise it with a mortar and pestle or food processor. Pour boiling water on to 1–5 g and drink daily.

Distinctive features: Fennel is one of the best remedies for physical weakness and lack of vitality due to insufficient or cold stomach energy, which stops the body from taking enough nutrients and energy out of the food.

SUO YANG

Latin name: Cynomortum coccinaum

Chinese name: Suo Yang

Botany: A fleshy plant with red-brown roots, full of scales and wrinkles

Found in: Mongolia and north and west China

Used parts of the plant: Roots and stem

The relevant organs: Kidneys, lungs and intestines

Energy: Warm

Flavour: Sweet

Effects: In traditional Chinese medicine Suo Yang tones the kidney Yin as well as kidney Yang and feeds the marrow. It serves as an aphrodisiac, stimulates, promotes the production of semen and relieves inflammation of the mucus membrane.

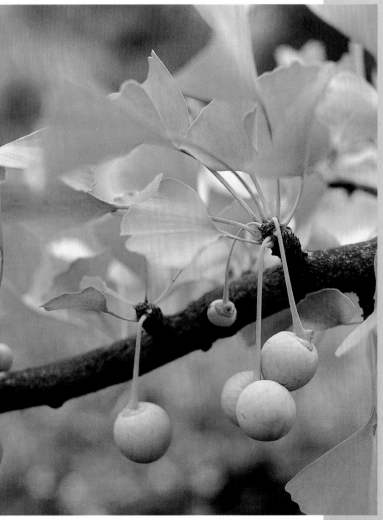

Areas of application: In traditional Chinese medicine, it is used for a lack of kidney energy, and for systems of inner dryness, premature ejaculation, pain in the back and knees, dry skin, dry mouth, thirst, constipation caused by dryness of the intestines.

Dosage: Brew 5–12 g and drink in two doses on an empty stomach

GINGKO SEEDS

Latin name: Gingko Biloba
Chinese name: Ying hsing
Botany: A tree reaching up to 35 m in height, with fan-shaped leaves and green-white buds, which open up during the night but drop very quickly; 1 to 2 cm long fruits with a smooth, hard, pale brown shell
Found in: China, Japan and by now also in Europe and in North America
Used parts of the plant: seeds
The relevant organs: Heart, kidneys and lungs
Energy: Neutral
Flavour: Sweet, bitter
Effects: In traditional Chinese medicine, Gingko stimulates the inherited energy, feeds the kidney Yin, warms the lung energy, it draws together and calms, alleviates coughs, strengthens the heart, stimulates digestion and serves as an antidote to alcohol poisoning.

Areas of application: Asthma, tuberculosis, coughs, bladder infection, gonorrhoea, painful and frequent urination, alcohol poisoning
Dosage: Brew 5–15 g and drink in 2 doses after meals

GINGKO ROOT

Latin name: Gingko Biloba
Chinese name: Bai guo gen
Botany: See Gingko seeds
Used parts of the plant: Root
The relevant organs: Kidneys
Energy: Neutral
Flavour: Sweet

Important

Large amounts of Gingko seeds can cause toxic reactions, for example, vomiting and cramps. A long-term application can cause a loss of appetite.

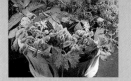

Effects: Stimulates and draws together.

Areas of application: Nocturnal emission, menstruation disturbances

Dosage: Brew 10–15 g and drink in 2 doses on an empty stomach.

Distinctive features: In contrast to the seeds, the roots of the Gingko tree are not toxic and can therefore be used for a longer period of time without concern.

GINSENG

Latin name: Panax ginseng

Chinese name: Ren shen

Botany: A perennial plant, which grows 60–80 cm high with a fleshy, split branch roots. It has a straight stem without branches and a pink flower. There is white and red ginseng, of the two, red Ginseng is more effective.

Found in: Northeast China, Manchuria, Korea, and Siberia

Used parts of the plant: Roots

The relevant organs: Spleen, lungs.

Energy: Warm

Flavour: Sweet, slightly bitter

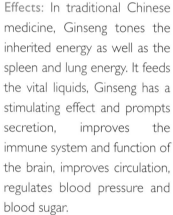

Effects: In traditional Chinese medicine, Ginseng tones the inherited energy as well as the spleen and lung energy. It feeds the vital liquids, Ginseng has a stimulating effect and prompts secretion, improves the immune system and function of the brain, improves circulation, regulates blood pressure and blood sugar.

Areas of application: In traditional Chinese medicine, it is used for lack of energy, a deficiency of lung and spleen energy, nervous exhaustion, loss of appetite, night sweats, cold extremities, for convalescence, memory loss, impotence, strokes, diabetes, raised or lowered blood pressure, blood deficiency, a pounding heart, suprarenal deficiency, weak immune system, inflammation of the stomach lining and morning sickness.

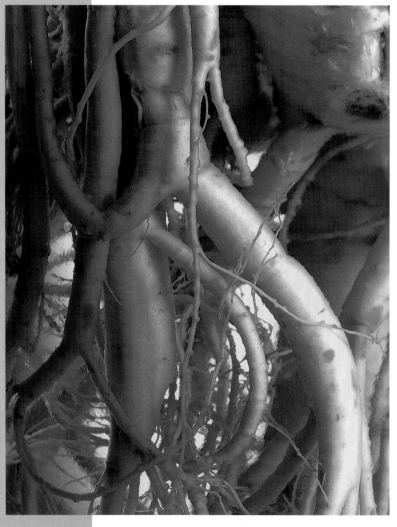

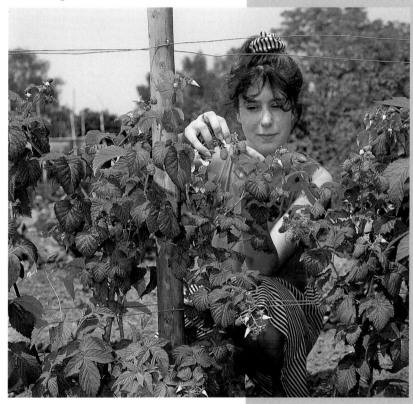

Dosage: Brew 5–10 g and drink in the morning, in one dose, on an empty stomach. (Boil in a pan for 30–60 minutes). For a tincture, allow 50–60 g of high-quality Ginseng to infuse in 1 litre of alcohol for 2–4 months. Take twice a day on an empty stomach.

Not to be used in the case of: Colds, pneumonia or lung infection

Incompatible with: Iron or other metal compounds and metal kitchen appliances, amethyst, milk products and tea

Distinctive Features: Ginseng is the most famous herb in Chinese medicine. Its reputation as a health tonic has also reached the Western Hemisphere. New studies have proved successful use of the herb in traditional Chinese medicine and have found other important areas where Ginseng can be used.

WILD ANGELICA

Latin name: Angelica villosa

Chinese name: Du huo

Botany: A trifoliate plant bearing umbels on thin stems; long vertical and horizontal stripes on the roots

Found in: Szechwan and other western provinces of China and Tibet

Used parts of the plant: Roots

The relevant organs: Kidneys and bladder

Energy: Slightly warm

Flavour: Spicy, bitter

Effects: According to traditional Chinese medicine, it eases inner heat, stimulates the sweat glands and relieves water retention through the skin, eases pain caused by rheumatic inflammation.

Areas of application: In traditional Chinese medicine, eases symptoms caused by wind, humidity, headaches, numbness, blurred vision, arthritis, rheumatism, numb extremities (caused by humidity), back and knee pain.

Dosage: Brew 3–6 g and drink in 2 doses on an empty stomach.

RASPBERRIES

Latin name: Rubus coreanus

Chinese name: Fu pen dze

Botany: A perenial plant with small thorns, sawed edges on the leaves and small red berries.

Found in: Mid and west China, Europe, a related species grows in North America

Used parts of the plant: The unripened fruits

The relevant organs: Kidney, liver

Energy: Slightly warm

Flavour: Sweet, sour

Effects: In traditional Chinese medicines; raspberries tone the kidneys- and liver-

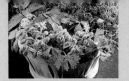

energy, stimulates the yang energy; has a general stimulating effect, draws together, prompts the semen production, improves vision

Areas of application: In traditional Chinese medicine, raspberries are used to treat: a lack of kidney- and liver-energy, impotence, male and female infertility, physical exhaustion, and incontinence as well as bed wetting in children.

Dosage: Brew 5–10 g and drink in two doses on an empty stomach. Tincture: infuse 50–60 g in 1 litre of alcohol for 1 to 2 months. Then drink 25 to 30 ml twice daily on an empty stomach.

To treat impotence Chinese herbal books recommend roasting unripened raspberries in a hot pan or oven, then pulverising them and taking 9g twice daily with a little alcohol.

COLTSFOOT

Latin name: Tussilago farfar
Chinese name: Kuan dung hua
Botany: This plant has a cotton wool like fuzz on the stems and underside of the leaves; it has large yellow flowers and horse shoe shaped leaves, the buds contain saponine, inucin, stearin and choline and tastes spicy.
Found in: North China, Europe, Africa, Siberia, and North America
Used part of the plant: Petals, buds, leaves
The relevant organs: Lungs
Energy: Warm

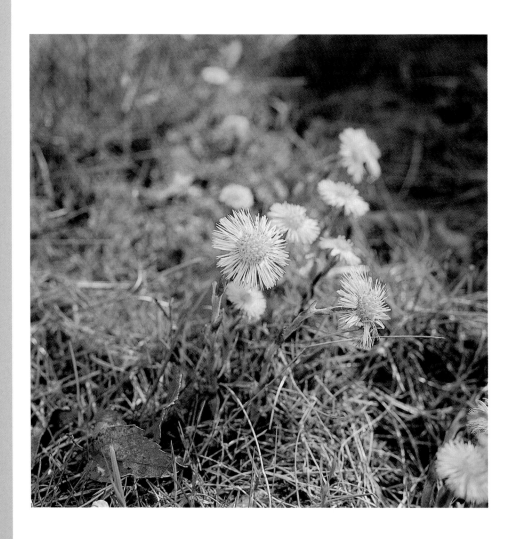

Flavour: Spicy

Effects: In traditional Chinese medicine, Coltsfoot tones the lung-energy, it eases coughs, prompts the body to cough out phlegm, stops swelling, relieves inflammations of the mucus membrane in the lungs.

Areas of application: In traditional Chinese medicine Coltsfoot helps with an empty lung-energy, coughs and smoking coughs, asthma, shortage of breath caused by a blockage in the lungs, acute and chronic lung-infections.

Dosage: Brew 5–12 g of petals and buds or 5–10 g of leaves and drink in 2 doses on an empty stomach. Leaves are mainly used for coughs and lung blockages.

Incompatible with: Glauber's salt and forsythia

Distinctive features: In China the leaves and petals are finely chopped and are smoked when someone has a chronic cough.

GINGER

Latin name: Zingiber officinale

Chinese name: Gan jiang

Botany: Similar to sugar cane, this plant reaches a height of about 1 metre. It has pointed leaves; the ends of the stalks are encased, fresh rootstock forms irregular, fleshy, yellow-brown tubers.

Found in: All tropical zones

Used parts of the plant: Dried rootstock

The relevant organs: Stomach, spleen, heart, lungs and kidneys.

Energy: Warm

Flavour: Spicy

Effects: In traditional Chinese medicine, Ginger stimulates the Yang energies, warms the lungs and stomach energy, it strengthens the stomach, prevents vomit-ing, stimulates the saliva flow, strengthens the heart and has a decongestive effect.

Areas of application: In traditional Chinese medicine, Ginger is used to treat a cold spleen, stomach and lung energy, lack of Yang energy, an emptiness of blood energy, nausea, vomiting, travel sickness, pain and coldness in the stomach, cold hands and feet, a cough with phlegm, stomach ulcers, colds, high cholesterol, and inflammation of the pancreas.

Dosage: Brew 10 g and drink in 2 doses on an empty stomach. Brown sugar is suitable for flavouring.

Not to be used in the case of: Pregnancy or high fever

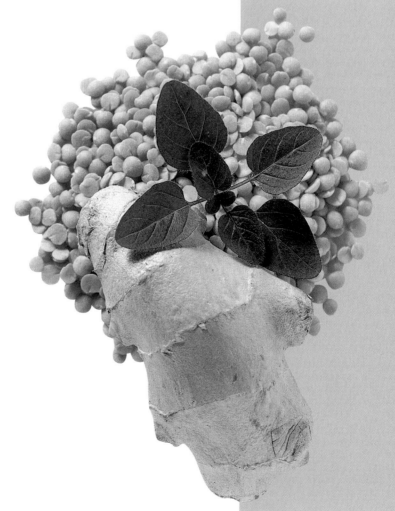

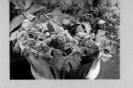
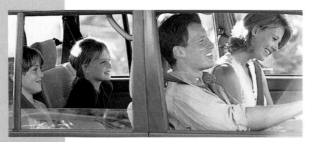

Ginger is a valued cure for travel sickness and has no unwanted side effects. Take 3 capsules, size 00 filled with pulverised dried ginger, a few hours before departure and then 2 capsules every hour or when necessary.

Distinctive features: In traditional Chinese medicine, fresh ginger is mainly used for fish poisoning as well as colds of the lung and stomach. As Ginger stimulates absorption of nutrients, it is often added to various remedies to help other herbs be more quickly absorbed and to strengthen their effect. Ginger contains a digestion-stimulating enzyme, zingibain the stimulating effect on the digestive system is stronger than that of the enzyme papain.

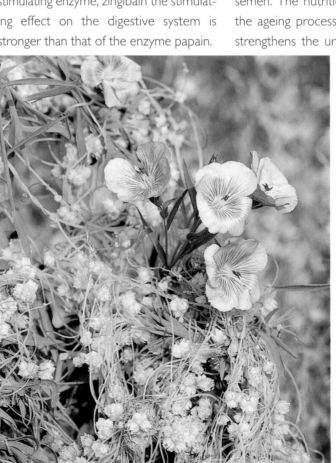

JAPANESE DODDER

Latin name: Cuscuta japonica

Chinese name: Tu seh dze

Botany: An annual parasitic plant with red-brown stalks and few leaves, brown seeds, with almost no smell or taste. Contains glykosid cuscutin.

Found in: Japan and China

Used parts of the plant: Seeds

Energy: Neutral

Flavour: Sweet and spicy

Effects: In traditional Chinese medicine, the Japanese Dodder tones the kidney as well as the liver energy and strengthens semen. The nutritious tonic slows down the ageing process, improves vision, and strengthens the urinary tract, bones and tendons.

Areas of application: In traditional Chinese medicine, when there is a lack of liver and kidney energy as well as symptoms of empty coldness, impotence, premature ejaculation, nocturnal emission, incontinence and premature ageing.

Dosage: Brew 7–12 g and drink in 2 doses on an empty stomach.

Not to be used in the case of: Open wounds and abscesses, not completely healed wounds; do not use the herb for longer than a month as this would slow down the healing process.

CARDAMOM

Latin name: Alpina oxyphylla
Chinese name: Yi jih ren
Botany: A stalky plant reaching the height of 2,50 m, the flower stems come directly out of the root, it has small fruits that grow like capsules on the stalk, these hold the precious seeds which are also used as a spice in cooking.
Found in: India, Malaysia, and South China
Used parts of the plant: Seeds
The relevant organs: Spleen, kidneys
Energy: Warm
Flavour: Spicy
Effects: According to traditional Chinese medicine cardamom tones the kidney-Yang, it feeds the bones and tendons, warms the kidneys and spleen, strengthens the stomach, disperses wind, draws together, helps prevent an unnecessary desire to urinate and keeps weak digestion under control.
Areas of application: In traditional Chinese medicine cardamom is put to use when there is cold-spleen and cold-kidney-symptoms, a lack of kidney-yang, vomiting and diarrhoea caused by inner cold, incontinence, diarrhoea, stomach ache, premature ejaculation, impotence and vomiting.
Dosage: Brew 3–10 g drink in 2 doses on an empty stomach
Not to be used in the case of: Stomach ulcers

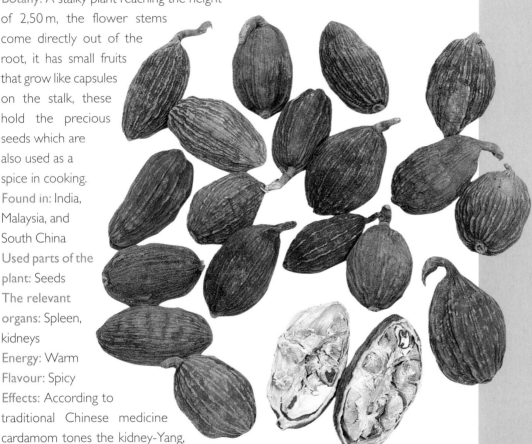

GARLIC

Latin name: Allium Sativum
Chinese name: Da suan
Botany: 15–30 cm high plants with cylindrical stalks. Lower part surrounded with leaves and a round tuber.
Found in: Worldwide. The remedies refer to the type found in China, Japan, Nepal, Tibet and Northern India.

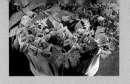

If a Cold Threatens

According to traditional Chinese medicine, to prevent a cold you should take 10 cloves of fresh garlic, peel and puree them then press the juice out through a cloth. Fill the juice into a small bottle and apply one drop into each nostril 3 times a day.

Important

Excessive amounts of garlic, is supposed to damage the eyes, cause numbness and scatter the energy. In traditional Chinese medicine this means that too much garlic causes raised fire energy.

Used parts of the plants: Tuber
The relevant organs: Stomach and large intestines
Energy: Warm
Flavour: Spicy
Effects: In traditional Chinese medicine, Garlic expels inner cold and inner dampness. It kills worms and parasites in the digestion tract and conducts them out of the body, kills bacteria and fungi, strengthens the stomach, stimulates and decongests, aids digestion, raises secretion in the stomach intestines and bronchial tubes, prevents tumour growth, lowers raised blood pressure.
Areas of application: In traditional Chinese medicine, Garlic is used to treat symptoms of inner cold, and inner dampness, tumours and swellings, tuberculosis, worms, and other parasites, diarrhoea, nose bleeds, bacterial infections, abscesses, high cholesterol, blocked arteries, raised blood pressure, colds, influenza, vaginal

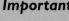

infections, candida, athletes foot, and other fungal infections.
Dosage: Internal: 3–5 fresh cloves a day,

raw with meals;
External: apply a puree of fresh garlic cloves on to abscesses; apply the puree generously to athletes foot, cover with a clean, dry cloth, remove the cloth after 1–2 hours and wipe away the remaining garlic (do not use water).
Incompatible with: Honey

WHITE CEDAR

Latin name: Thuja orientalis
Chinese name: Bo dze ren
Botany: Pyramid shaped fir-tree with small scaly needles and nutritious fruits
Found in: China, Japan and India
Used parts of the plant: Seeds
The relevant organs: Heart, spleen and liver
Energy: Neutral
Flavour: Sweet and spicy
Effects: In traditional Chinese medicine, the white cedar strengthens the heart energy, supports the spleen and feeds the liver, it calms, it softens tissue in the large intestines and stimulates the production of semen.
Areas of application: Sleeplessness, pounding heart, constipation physical weakness, poor diet, and male infertility.

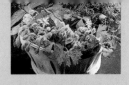

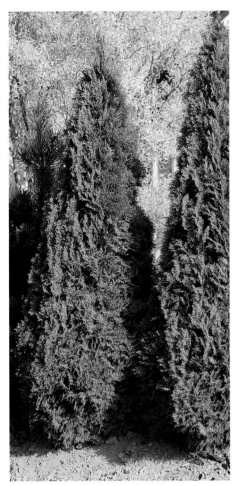

Dosage: Brew 5–10 g and drink in 2 doses on an empty stomach.

LOTUS SEEDS

Latin name: Nelumbium nucifera

Chinese name: Lien dze

Botany: A perennial water plant, with thick edible, starchy roots. It has large round leaves and a crown of leaves surrounding the flower and petals in various shades of pink and white.

Found in: Tropical regions of Asia and Australia.

Used parts of the plant: Seeds

The relevant organs: Spleen, kidneys, heart

Energy: Neutral

Flavour: Sweet

Effects: In traditional Chinese medicine, Lotus seeds tone the heart and spleen energies and feed the semen, they stimulate, are styptic and strengthen the nervous system.

Areas of application: In traditional Chinese medicine, Lotus seeds are used when a lack of heart and kidney energy arises, for impotence, nocturnal emission, menstruation problems, sleeplessness, sexual diseases, diarrhoea, a weak heart as well as inflammation of the pancreas.

Dosage: Brew 6–12 g and drink in 3 doses on an empty stomach. Powder (pure, capsules, pills or paste) take 4–8 g in 3 doses on an empty stomach.

Not to be used in the case of: Constipation, digestion problems, wind.

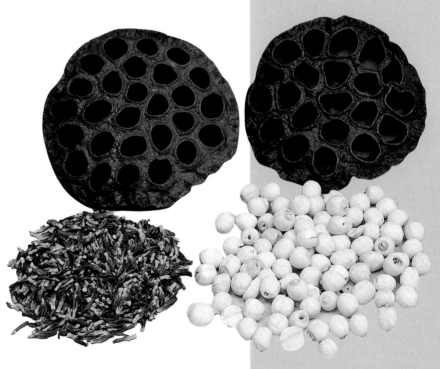

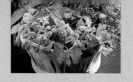

If you are collecting dandelion yourself, take the whole plant including the roots, remove the soil and dry in the sun and wind, store in a dry place. Dandelion does not only belong to medicinal herbs, but is also a nutritious food. The leaves contain lots of vitamin A, B and C as well as a lot of minerals. Dandelion leaves are a tasty and nutritious ingredient to salads and soups. To take away the bitter taste, place them in salty water for 30 minutes or blanch them shortly in boiling water.

DANDELIONS

Latin name: Tarataraxacum officinale
Chinese name: Pu gung Ying
Botany: A perennial plant with bright green jagged leaves and yellow petals, it flowers from April to November, a milky liquid seeps from the roots and stem
Used part of the plant: The whole plant
The relevant organs: Liver, stomach
Energy: Cold
Flavour: Bitter, sweet
Effects: In traditional Chinese medicine dandelion eliminates inner heat, works as an antidote, raises bile production, stimulates the production of milk, Strengthens the stomach functions, lowers fever and swelling, removes blood clots and cleans the blood.

Areas of application: In traditional Chinese medicine dandelion is used for symptoms of inner heat, food poisoning, painful and/or swollen breasts, breast tumours, blockage and inflammation of the liver and gallbladder, blood clots in the lungs and snake bites.
Dosage: For liver and gallbladder complaints and the connected strain, nausea and irritability brew 6–8 plants and drink in 2 doses on an empty stomach for 10–14 days. For a lack of lactation brew 10 plants and drink in 3 doses on an empty stomach. For breast tumours and the related pain and swelling brew 20 plants and drink in 3 doses on an empty stomach. Externally the juice of the plant can be used as an antidote for snakebites.

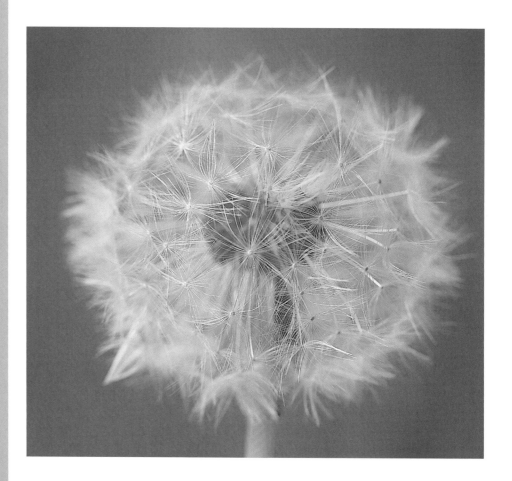

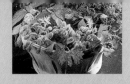

Distinctive features: In traditional Chinese medicine dandelion, because of its properties to stop swelling and blockages is an important treatment for the female sexual organs especially the breasts.

MINT

Latin name: Mentha arvensis

Chinese name: Bo he

Botany: A perennial plant 10–60 cm tall with erect stems, oval leaves with jagged edges and grape-shaped pink coloured flowers

Found in: Mint grows wild but is also cultivated in China, Southeast Asia, India and Europe.

Used parts of the plant: Leaves and delicate stems

The relevant organs: Lungs and liver

Energy: Cool

Flavour: Spicy

Effects: In traditional Chinese medicine, mint eliminates inner heat, expels wind heat, strengthens the stomach, eases wind, relieves water retention through the skin, eases pains and strengthens the nervous system.

Areas of application: In traditional Chinese medicine, mint treats symptoms of inner heat, headaches, coughs, sore throats, ear-ache, menstruation problems, digestive disorders and wind.

Dosage: Brew 2–4 g and drink in 1 dose on an empty stomach.

Tea infusion: Pour hot water over 1 g of powder and leave to infuse, drink on an

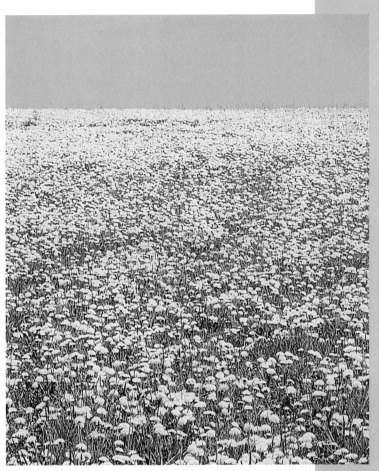

empty stomach. Sweeten the tea with a little honey if necessary.

Ointment: mix some mint powder with yellow Vaseline, almond oil, lanolin or with another grease base; apply the cooling and easing ointment to head, chest, stomach or other painful, blocked or inflamed areas.

Not to be used in the case of: Strong shivers or nervous exhaustion

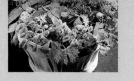

JIH MU

Latin name: Anemarrhena asphodeloides
Chinese name: Jih mu
Botany: A lily plant with a rootstock, which is covered with yellow or red hair. The petals are purplish on the inside and yellow on the outside. The herb tastes bitter but has a pleasant scent.

Found in: The mountains of north Peking and in most northern provinces of China
Used parts of plant: The rootstock and stalks
The relevant organs: Kidneys, lungs and stomach
Energy: Cold
Flavour: Bitter
Effects: According to traditional Chinese Medicine, the herb feeds the kidney-Yin and eliminates inner heat. It lowers fever, eases inflammation of the mucus membrane, softens irritated intestine tissue, activates the bladder and stops swelling.
Areas of application: Nocturnal emission, night sweats, impotence, weak erections caused by weakness in the suprarenal glands, diarrhoea, constipation, thirst, sleeplessness and irritability caused by too much inner heat, lung infections and bronchitis.
Dosage: Brew 6–12 g and drink 2 doses on an empty stomach. Powder: (pure capsules or pills) 5–10 g drink with warm water or wine in 2 doses on an empty stomach.
Not to be used in the case of: According to traditional Chinese medicine, empty-cold-conditions in the spleen and stomach and watery diarrhoea.
Distinctive Features: Chronic use can cause intestine lethargy.
Incompatible with: Iron preparations and objects made of iron.

BLACK PEPPER

Latin name: Piper nigrum
Chinese name: Hu jiao
Botany: A woody climbing plant with air roots and wild foliage, strong scented grey-black fruits
Found in: Indonesia, Hainen island in south China
Used parts of the plant: Dried unripened fruits
The relevant organs: Spleen, stomach
Energy: Hot
Flavour: Spicy
Effects: According to traditional Chinese medicine black pepper drives out blockages in the stomach which are caused by damp cold in the digestive tract, it

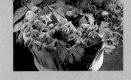

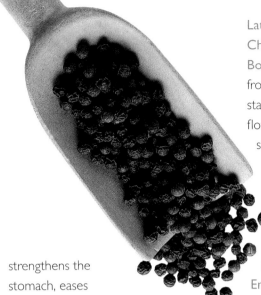

SOAPWORT

Latin Name: Saponaria vaccaria
Chinese Name: Wang bu liu hsing
Botany: An annual plant, which grows from 30 to 60 cm in height. It has erect stalks, long leaves and pink, bell-shaped flowers, cylindrical calyx with seed capsules, round, red-brown seeds, tastes bitter, contains saponin.
Found in: Western Asia southern Europe and China
Used parts of the plant: Seeds
The relevant organs: Liver and stomach
Energy: Neutral
Flavour: Bitter, sweet
Effects: In traditional Chinese medicine, soapwort stimulates the meridian (acupressure points); styptic, draws together, eases pain, has a mild laxative effect, stimulates the forming of milk, and regulates

strengthens the stomach, eases wind, stimulates the stomach lining, helps fight fish and meat poisoning.

Areas of application: According to traditional Chinese medicine black pepper is applied when damp cold arises in the spleen and stomach, it is also used for cold in the intestines, weak digestion, watery vomit, food poisoning (fish and meat), obesity, blocked sinuses.

Dosage: Brew 1, 5–3 g of herbs and drink in 2 doses 30–40 minutes after meals.

Not to be used in the case of: Inflammation of the digestive tract

Distinctive features: To balance out the cold Yin-energy, salads made of fresh raw vegetables can be generously flavoured with black pepper, the hot Yang-herb.

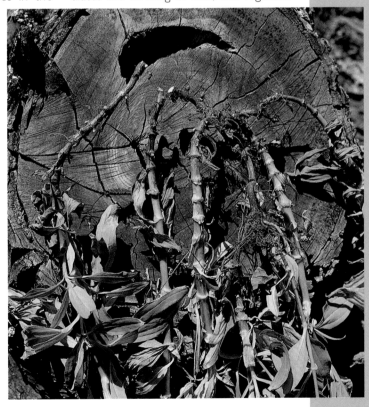

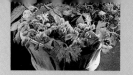

menstruation, eases coughs with phlegm.

Areas of application: Stroke, numb extremities, bleeding wounds, abscesses, chronic coughs, lactation deficiency, headaches

Dosage: Externally: apply pulverised herb directly to wounds, abscesses, to stop bleeding and to accelerate the healing process.

Internally: brew 5–7 g and drink in 2 doses before or after meals.

(Warning: the herb tastes bitter!)

Not to be used: In pregnancy

LIQUORICE

Latin name: Glycrrhiza uralensis

Chinese name: Gan tsao

Botany: Perennial plant with erect stalks, small oval leaves, arranged in a grape formation. Purple-red petals, roots are grey-brown or dark brown outside and yellow inside tastes noticeably sweeter than sugar cane.

Found in: Northern China, Mongolia, Siberia, central Asia.

Used parts of the plant: Roots

The relevant organs: All twelve organs

Energy: Neutral

Flavour: Sweet

Effects: In traditional Chinese medicine, liquorice tones the spleen and stomach energy, it represses the heart-fire, and it cures external cold; acts as a decongestant, eases inflammations of the mucus membrane the lungs and the bronchial tubes, stimulates, lowers fever, has a slight laxative

effect, calms, eases coughs, lowers a raised cholesterol and blood sugar and prevents tumour growth.

Well Known and Popular

Liquorice is highly regarded in traditional Chinese Medicine and is often used in Chinese herbal medicine. Numerous remedies include liquorice. It improves the taste of other herbs and extends their effect.

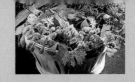

Areas of application: Colds, fever, sore throats, blockages in the lungs and bronchial tubes, stomach ulcers, inflammation of the stomach lining, excessive gastric acid, diabetes, gallbladder infection, irritability, alcohol and medicine poisoning, hepatitis, cirrhosis of the liver and skin irritations.

SZECHUAN PEPPER

Latin name: Zanthoxylum piperitum
Chinese name: Chuan jiao
Botany: Small, deciduous tree, with dark brown thorny bark, hard shiny leaves and spicy tasting fruits, which contain black, shining seeds

Used part of the plant: Fruits, fruit leaves and seeds
The relevant organs: Kidneys, spleen
Energy: Hot
Flavour: Spicy, bitter
Effects: In traditional Chinese medicine, the pepper expels dampness, it scatters cold, strengthens the stomach, acts as a diuretic, relieves wind and warms.
Areas of application: Food blockage in digestion tract, frequent urination, and bladder infections
Dosage: Brew 2–5 g and drink in 2 doses before or after meals
Not to be used in the case of: Pregnancy

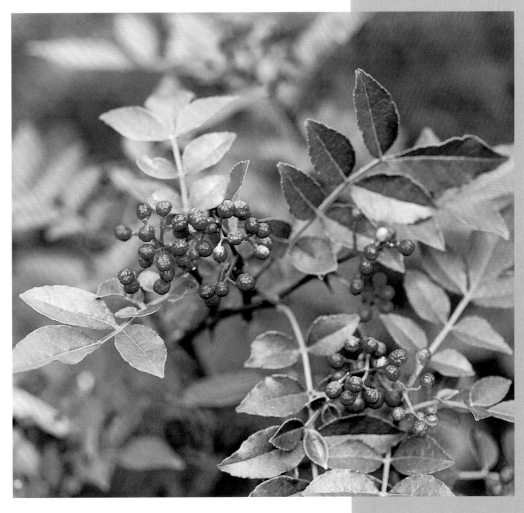

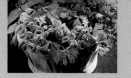

CINNAMON

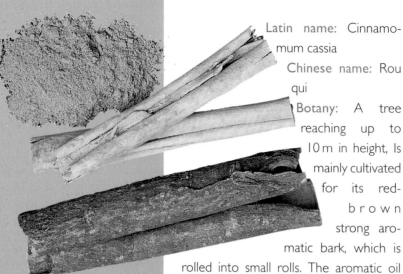

Latin name: Cinnamomum cassia

Chinese name: Rou qui

Botany: A tree reaching up to 10 m in height, Is mainly cultivated for its red-brown strong aromatic bark, which is rolled into small rolls. The aromatic oil contains up to 80 % cinnamon aldehyde.

Found in: Southern China, Vietnam, Laos and Sumatra

Used parts of the plant: Untreated bark taken from old, mature trees

The relevant organs: Liver, spleen, and kidneys

Energy: Very hot

Flavour: Spicy, sweet

Effects: According to traditional Chinese medicine cinnamon tones the Yang-energies and warms, it strengthens the stomach, eases pain, draws together, stimulates the forming of sweat and releases water retention through the skin, improves vision and stimulates the circulation.

Areas of application: In traditional Chinese medicine a lack of kidney- and spleen-yang, as well as inner cold in the stomach, are indications to use cinnamon, which is also used for lack of appetite, tiredness, stomach ache, lack of energy after a long illness or operation, irregular or painful menstruation, red, swollen eyes and extremities.

Doses: Brew 2–5 g and drink in 2 doses on an empty stomach. If you wish to make the effects stronger add 2 g of liquorice root and 3 slices of ginseng to the brew.

Incompatible with: Onions and kaolin

Distinctive features: In traditional Chinese medicine cinnamon is a great supplement for many other herbs, especially for Yang-tonics. It strengthens the warming and toning characteristics of herbal tinctures and improves their taste. Cinnamon is considered one of the strongest warming agents in traditional Chinese medicine. It warms cold extremities and the inner organs.

TWO SIMPLE EXAMPLES OF HERBAL REMEDIES

A GINSENG BREW FOR A LOWERED STOMACH (REN SHEN RANG)

You will find this classical remedy in many Chinese herb books. It is still used in its original form today.

The unusual lowering of the stomach in the lower abdominal manifests itself as a loose, flacid stomach lining. The stomach lining no longer posseses the usual tension and movement. This means that the undigested food is not transported further, which causes digestion problems such as burping, nausea, and wind.

Ginseng is used in this recipe as a stimulant for the digestion. It warms the stomach, raises stomach juice secretion, activates stomach lining cells and is responsible for returning the digestive system back to normal.

Application: Lowered stomach, characterised by a bloated upper abdominal, indigestion, deep burping, stomach-ache, nausea, loss of appetite, weak digestion and constipation.

Ingredients:

Ginseng	3 g
Liquorice	3 g
Atractylis ovata	3 g
Ginger (dried)	3 g

Brew: drink in 2 doses on an empty stomach

CINNAMON AND GINSENG BREW FOR HEADACHES (GUI JI REN SHEN RANG)

This is a favourite classical remedy for tension headaches and migraines. According to clinical experiment in China, this remedy has a positive effect on around 50 % of all patients with chronic tension headaches.

Application: Headaches and migraines with accompanying symptoms such as nausea, blocked feelings in the chest and/or the solar plexus (the latter is a complex nerve network made up of vegetative nerves, which is found in the stomach area; a hard punch can irritate so strongly that it can cause a shock)

Ingredients:

Cinnamon	4 g
Liquorice	3 g
Atractylis ovate	3 g
Ginseng	2 g
Ginger (dried)	1 g

Brew: drink 2 doses mornings and evening on an empty stomach

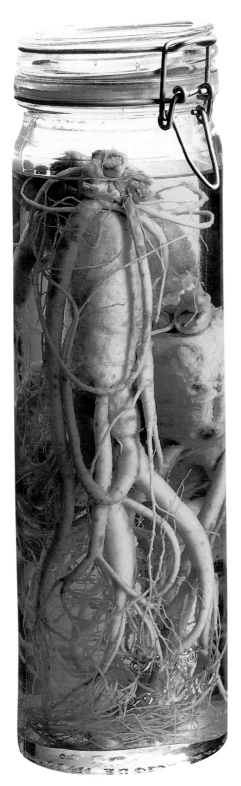

Ginseng (see page 46 f.) is one of the few plants that have become very popular in Great Britain. It contains resin, saponin, tannic and bitter substances, many minerals and trace elements as well as panazen. Saponin influences the sugar metabolism, while panazen influences the heart and circulation.

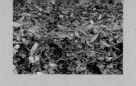

RELEVANT ADDRESSES FOR CHINESE MEDICINAL HERBS

Chinese chemists have become more popular in Great Britain over the years, but you can also obtain medicinal herbs from your local chemists. If your local chemist does not supply the required herbs, here are a few addresses to help you in your search. Some of the companies listed here also deliver ready-made mixtures.

Accupuncture and Herbal Medicine
Sino Medica
92 Didsbury Road
Stockport
SK4 2JL
www.acupunctures.co.uk

Birmingham Centre
for Chinese Medicine
245 Alcester Road South
Kings Heath
Birmingham
B14 6DT
www.bccm.freeserve.co.uk

International Register of Consultant
Herbalists and Homeopaths
32 King Edwards Road
Swansea
South Wales
SA1 4CC
www.irch.org

National Institution of Medical Herbalists
56 Longbrook Street
Exeter
Devon
EX4 6AH
www.nimh.org.uk

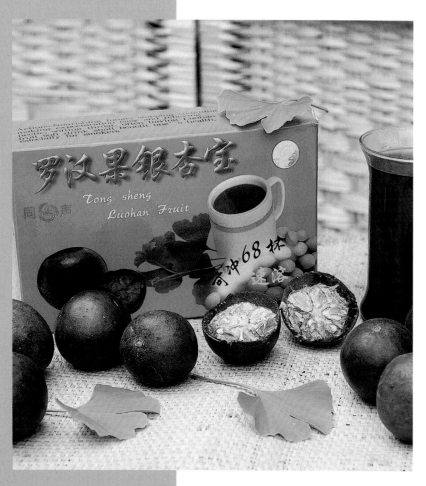

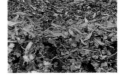

INDEX

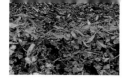

INDEX